Kalliope Nina Diakopoulos

Role of autophagy in pancreatic disease

Kalliope Nina Diakopoulos

Role of autophagy in pancreatic disease

Südwestdeutscher Verlag für Hochschulschriften

Impressum / Imprint
Bibliografische Information der Deutschen Nationalbibliothek: Die Deutsche Nationalbibliothek verzeichnet diese Publikation in der Deutschen Nationalbibliografie; detaillierte bibliografische Daten sind im Internet über http://dnb.d-nb.de abrufbar.
Alle in diesem Buch genannten Marken und Produktnamen unterliegen warenzeichen-, marken- oder patentrechtlichem Schutz bzw. sind Warenzeichen oder eingetragene Warenzeichen der jeweiligen Inhaber. Die Wiedergabe von Marken, Produktnamen, Gebrauchsnamen, Handelsnamen, Warenbezeichnungen u.s.w. in diesem Werk berechtigt auch ohne besondere Kennzeichnung nicht zu der Annahme, dass solche Namen im Sinne der Warenzeichen- und Markenschutzgesetzgebung als frei zu betrachten wären und daher von jedermann benutzt werden dürften.

Bibliographic information published by the Deutsche Nationalbibliothek: The Deutsche Nationalbibliothek lists this publication in the Deutsche Nationalbibliografie; detailed bibliographic data are available in the Internet at http://dnb.d-nb.de.
Any brand names and product names mentioned in this book are subject to trademark, brand or patent protection and are trademarks or registered trademarks of their respective holders. The use of brand names, product names, common names, trade names, product descriptions etc. even without a particular marking in this work is in no way to be construed to mean that such names may be regarded as unrestricted in respect of trademark and brand protection legislation and could thus be used by anyone.

Coverbild / Cover image: www.ingimage.com

Verlag / Publisher:
Südwestdeutscher Verlag für Hochschulschriften
ist ein Imprint der / is a trademark of
OmniScriptum GmbH & Co. KG
Heinrich-Böcking-Str. 6-8, 66121 Saarbrücken, Deutschland / Germany
Email: info@svh-verlag.de

Herstellung: siehe letzte Seite /
Printed at: see last page
ISBN: 978-3-8381-5061-1

Zugl. / Approved by: München, TU, Diss., 2014

Copyright © 2015 OmniScriptum GmbH & Co. KG
Alle Rechte vorbehalten. / All rights reserved. Saarbrücken 2015

1 ZUSAMMENFASSUNG

Ziel der vorliegenden Doktorarbeit war es die Bedeutung der Autophagie im Pankreas zu untersuchen. Autophagie beschreibt einen homöostatischen Mechanismus, der für die Regulation von Zellmetabolismus und Zellüberleben wichtig ist. Defekte in Autophagie wurden bereits in multiplen Erkrankungen beschrieben. Studien haben auch eine Rolle der Autophagie in Pankreatitis detektiert, aber die bisherigen Ergebnisse lassen noch keine Schlussfolgerungen zu.

Um die Bedeutung der Autophagie für die exokrine Pankreasphysiologie aufzuklären, wurden Mäuse mit pankreasspezifischer, genetischer Inaktivierung von *Atg5* im Detail charakterisiert. Behandlungen mit spezifischen Diäten wurden vollzogen, um den Effekt von Diätkompositionen und Antioxidantien auf die Phänotypentwicklung zu untersuchen. Schließlich wurde der murine Pankreasphänotyp mit Pankreata von Patienten mit chronischer Pankreatitis (CP) auf Gemeinsamkeiten verglichen.

Pankreasspezifische Inaktivierung der Atg5-abhängigen Autophagie in Mäusen resultierte in atropher CP, mit einer signifikant höheren Frequenz in männlichen Mäusen. Verlust von *Atg5* führte zu Entzündung, Nekrose, azinärer-duktaler Metaplasie und Hypertrophie der Azinuszellen. Pankreasatrophie und Degeneration folgten. Analysen des Transkriptoms und Metaboloms legten exzessiven oxidativen Stress und insuffiziente Glutamat-abhängige metabolische Signalwege als Phänotypdeterminanten dar. Verlust der Autophagie führte ebenfalls zur Akkumulation von p62, dilatiertem endoplasmatischen Retikulum, und geschädigten Mitochondrien, verschlimmert durch einen p62/Nqo1/p53-gesteuerten Signalweg. Eine starke Erschwerung des Verlaufs experimenteller akuter Pankreatitis konnte ebenfalls beschrieben werden, was auf eine Beeinträchtigung der Stressresistenz von Azinuszellen hindeutet. Bemerkenswerterweise konnten Antioxidantien, insbesondere in Kombination mit Fettsäuren aus Palmöl, die Progression zu CP und exokriner Pankreasatrophie verhindern. Zudem konnten viele morphologische und biochemische Ähnlichkeiten mit humaner CP beschrieben werden.

Demnach wird hier das erste genetische Mausmodell humaner CP präsentiert. Außerdem wird durch die Anwendung einer spezifischen diätischen Zusammensetzung mit vielversprechenden therapeutischen Ergebnissen dessen klinische Relevanz hervorgehoben.

Part of this thesis was submitted for publication and was under revision at the time of thesis submission. The final accepted publication is:

Kalliope N. Diakopoulos, Marina Lesina, Sonja Wörmann, Liang Song, Michaela Aichler, Lorenz Schild, Anna Artati, Werner Römisch-Margl, Thomas Wartmann, Robert Fischer, Yashar Kabiri, Hans Zischka, Walter Halangk, Ihsan Ekin Demir, Claudia Pilsak, Axel Walch, Christos S. Mantzoros, Jörg M. Steiner, Mert Erkan, Roland M. Schmid, Heiko Witt, Jerzy Adamski and Hana Algül. Impaired Autophagy Induces Chronic Atrophic Pancreatitis in Mice via Sex- and Nutrition-Dependent Processes. Gastroenterology. 2015 Mar;148(3):626-638.e17. doi: 10.1053/j.gastro.2014.12.003. Epub 2014 Dec 11. PMID 25497209

Additional publications not related to this thesis include:

Moon HS, Chamberland JP, **Diakopoulos KN**, Fiorenza CG, Ziemke F, Schneider B, Mantzoros CS. Leptin and amylin act in an additive manner to activate overlapping signaling pathways in peripheral tissues; in vitro and ex vivo studies in humans. Diabetes Care. 2011 Jan;34(1):132-8. doi: 10.2337/dc10-0518. Epub 2010 Sep 24. PMID 20870968

Aronis KN, **Diakopoulos KN**, Fiorenza CG, Chamberland JP, Mantzoros CS. Leptin administered in physiological or pharmacological doses does not regulate circulating angiogenesis factors in humans. Diabetologia. 2011 Sep;54(9):2358-67. doi: 10.1007/s00125-011-2201-x. Epub 2011 Jun 10. PMID 21660636

Mitsiades N, Pazaitou-Panayiotou K, Aronis KN, Moon HS, Chamberland JP, Liu X, **Diakopoulos KN**, Kyttaris V, Panagiotou V, Mylvaganam G, Tseleni-Balafouta S, Mantzoros CS. Circulating adiponectin is inversely associated with risk of thyroid cancer: in vivo and in vitro studies. J Clin Endocrinol Metab. 2011 Dec;96(12):E2023-8. doi: 10.1210/jc.2010-1908. Epub 2011 Sep 21. PMID 21937620

Dalamaga M, **Diakopoulos KN**, Mantzoros CS. The role of adiponectin in cancer: a review of current evidence. Endocr Rev. 2012 Aug;33(4):547-94. doi: 10.1210/er.2011-1015. Epub 2012 Apr 30. PMID 22547160

Moon HS, Liu X, Nagel JM, Chamberland JP, **Diakopoulos KN**, Brinkoetter MT, Hatziapostolou M, Wu Y, Robson SC, Iliopoulos D, Mantzoros CS. Salutary effects of adiponectin on colon cancer: in vivo and in vitro studies in mice. Gut. 2013 Apr;62(4):561-70. doi: 10.1136/gutjnl-2012-302092. Epub 2012 Jun 26. PMID 22735569

Neuhöfer P, Liang S, Einwächter H, Schwerdtfeger C, Wartmann T, Treiber M, Zhang H, Schulz HU, Dlubatz K, Lesina M, **Diakopoulos KN**,

Wörmann S, Halangk W, Witt H, Schmid RM, Algül H. Deletion of IκBα activates RelA to reduce acute pancreatitis in mice through up-regulation of Spi2A. Gastroenterology. 2013 Jan;144(1):192-201. doi: 10.1053/j.gastro.2012.09.058. Epub 2012 Oct 3. PMID 23041330

Schiller C, Huber JE, **Diakopoulos KN**, Weiss EH. Tunneling nanotubes enable intercellular transfer of MHC class I molecules. Hum Immunol. 2013 Apr;74(4):412-6. doi: 10.1016/j.humimm.2012.11.026. Epub 2012 Dec 7. PMID 23228397

Schiller C, **Diakopoulos KN**, Rohwedder I, Kremmer E, von Toerne C, Ueffing M, Weidle UH, Ohno H, Weiss EH. LST1 promotes the assembly of a molecular machinery responsible for tunneling nanotube formation. J Cell Sci. 2013 Feb 1;126(Pt 3):767-77. doi: 10.1242/jcs.114033. Epub 2012 Dec 13. PMID 23239025

Wörmann SM, **Diakopoulos KN**, Lesina M, Algül H. The immune network in pancreatic cancer development and progression. Oncogene. 2014 Jun 5;33(23):2956-67. doi: 10.1038/onc.2013.257. Epub 2013 Jul 15. PMID 23851493

Schiller C, Nowak C, **Diakopoulos KN**, Weidle UH, Weiss EH. An upstream open reading frame regulates LST1 expression during monocyte differentiation. PLoS One. 2014 May 9;9(5):e96245. doi: 10.1371/journal.pone.0096245. eCollection 2014. PMID 24816991

Parts of this thesis were presented at the following scientific meetings:

1) "Pankreasspezifische Inaktivierung der Atg5-abhängigen Autophagie führt zur Ausbildung einer chronisch atrophen Pankreatitis", *scientific presentation*
Nina Diakopoulos, Marina Lesina, Hans Zischka, Walter Halangk, Roland M Schmid, Heiko Witt, Michaela Aichler, Hana Algül

(Jahrestagung der Deutschen Gesellschaft für Verdauungs- und Stoffwechselkrankheiten, September 11th -14th 2013, Nuremberg, Germany)

2) "Pankreasspezifische Inaktivierung der Atg5-abhängigen Autophagie führt zur Ausbildung einer chronisch atrophen Pankreatitis", *scientific presentation*
Nina Diakopoulos, Marina Lesina, Hans Zischka, Walter Halangk, Roland M Schmid, Heiko Witt, Michaela Aichler, Hana Algül

(Jahrestagung des Deutschen Pankreasclubs, January 23rd – 25th 2014, Mannheim, Germany)

3) "Inactivation of autophagy in the pancreas induces chronic atrophic pancreatitis", *scientific poster presentation*
K.N. Diakopoulos, M. Lesina, W. Halangk, T. Wartmann, L. Schild, H. Zischka, M. Aichler, J. Adamski, H. Witt, C.S. Mantzoros, R. M. Schmid, H. Algül

(Keystone Symposium "Autophagy: Fundamentals to Disease", May 23rd to 28th 2014, Austin, TX)

2 TABLE OF CONTENT

1 ZUSAMMENFASSUNG 1
2 TABLE OF CONTENT 7
3 INTRODUCTION 11
  3.1 **Autophagy** 11
    3.1.1 Mechanism of autophagy 11
    3.1.2 Autophagy function 14
    3.1.3 Autophagy and disease 15
    3.1.4 P62: more than an autophagic adaptor protein 17
  3.2 **Pancreas** 20
    3.2.1 Morphology and function 20
    3.2.2 Pancreatic Pathology 21
  3.3 **Pancreas and autophagy** 23
  3.4 **Aim** 25
4 MATERIALS AND METHODS 26
  4.1 **Mice** 26
    4.1.1 Mouse models 26
    4.1.2 Acute pancreatitis 27
    4.1.3 Dietary modifications 28
    4.1.4 Induction of *ElastaseCre* expression 28
    4.1.5 Glucose Measurement and Intraperitoneal Glucose Tolerance Test (IPGTT) 28
  4.2 **DNA/RNA studies** 29
    4.2.1 Mouse genotyping 29
    4.2.2 RNA extraction 31
    4.2.3 cDNA synthesis 31
    4.2.4 Quantitative real time PCR analysis 31
    4.2.5 Detection of unspliced and spliced *Xbp1* 33
    4.2.6 Agarose gel electrophoresis 34
    4.2.7 Microarray analysis 34

4.2.8 *Atg5* exon sequencing in humans with CP 35
4.3 **Histology** 37
4.3.1 Tissue sections 37
4.3.2 Haematoxylin and eosin (H&E) staining 38
4.3.3 Immunohistochemistry 38
4.3.4 Co-immunofluorescence 40
4.3.5 Detection of GFP-LC3 puncta 41
4.3.6 Detection of Cre-Recombinase expression 41
4.3.7 Detection of Reactive Oxygen Species (ROS) 41
4.3.8 Quantification of relative acinar cell area 42
4.3.9 Quantification of proliferation (BrdU) and apoptosis (cleaved caspase 3) 42
4.3.10 Transmission Electron microscopy (TEM) 43
4.3.11 Human chronic pancreatitis samples 44
4.4 **Proteinbiochemistry** 44
4.4.1 Serum amylase and lipase measurement 44
4.4.2 Pancreatic tissue enzyme content and activity 45
4.4.3 Subcellular fractionation by isopycnic Percoll density centrifugation and measurement of GLDH activity 46
4.4.4 Mitochondrial Respiratory Complex II and IV Activity Assays in isolated pancreatic mitochondria 46
4.4.5 Protein extraction and quantification 48
4.4.6 SDS-PAGE 49
4.4.7 Western blot 50
4.5 **Metabolomics and Lipidomics** 52
4.5.1 Non-targeted metabolomics profiling 52
4.5.2 Characterization of mitochondrial cardiolipin composition 54
4.6 **Statistics** 56
5 **RESULTS** 57
5.1 **Autophagy in the pancreas** 57
5.1.1 Baseline and starvation induced autophagy 57

5.1.2 Acute pancreatitis and autophagy 58
5.2 Pancreas-specific inactivation of autophagy 58
5.2.1 *A5* mice exhibit features of CP 58
5.2.2 Adult acinar cells are resistant to autophagy deficiency 63
5.2.3 Persistent acinar-to-ductal metaplasia in *A5* mice 65
5.2.4 Whole genome transcriptomics and non-targeted metabolomics 67
5.2.5 ER stress, ROS and mitochondrial damage in *A5* mice 74
5.3 Role of p53 and p62 in pancreas-specific autophagy deficiency 79
5.4 Influence of gender 83
5.5 Induction of acute pancreatitis 86
5.6 Influence of diet 87
5.7 Similarities with human chronic pancreatitis 93

6 DISCUSSION 98
6.1 Impaired pancreatic autophagy induces chronic atrophic CP 99
6.2 Defective mitochondria cause ROS accumulation and subsequent metabolic deficiencies in pancreata of *A5* mice 101
6.3 The p62/Nrf2/Nqo1/p53 feed forward loop 103
6.4 The impact of gender and nutrition in regulating Atg5-dependent pathophysiology 104
6.5 Mice deficient in pancreatic autophagy: a new model for human CP 106

7 SUMMARY 108
8 REFERENCES 110
9 ABBREVIATIONS 119
10 ACKNOWLEDGEMENTS 120

3 INTRODUCTION

3.1 Autophagy

The term autophagy stems from the Greek word „*Auto-phagia*", meaning „self-eating". It was originally used for a process discovered by electron microscopy in the late 1950s by Christian de Duve[4]. Thus, autophagy is an intracellular degradation pathway employing lysosomes and targeting multiple cytoplasmic substrates such as protein aggregates and organelles. Autophagy can be separated into macroautophagy, microautophagy, and chaperone-mediated autophagy[5]. In this thesis, only macroautophagy (hereafter referred to as autophagy) will be analyzed.

3.1.1 Mechanism of autophagy

Autophagy starts with a double membrane vesicle termed autophagosome (Figure 1). Formation of autophagosomes is based on the concerted action of multiple Atg (i.e., autophagy related) proteins. Thus far, 37 *Atg* genes have been identified in yeast, less than half of which are involved in canonical autophagy. Canonical autophagy is highly conserved among organisms, including mammals. In mammals the core autophagy machinery is made up of 29 *Atg* genes[4].

Various intracellular signals regulate autophagy initiation (see 3.1.2). ER-mitochondrial contact sites have been suggested to act as sites of autophagosome formation, with additional contributions from the Golgi apparatus, endosomes, and the plasma membrane. During initiation, two protein complexes named ULK and Beclin-1/class III PI3K localize at the site of autophagosome formation, phosphorylating downstream targets, and generating a pool of phosphatidyl-inositol-3-phosphate (PI3P). PI3P-accumulation recruits additional Atg and PI3P-effector proteins, mediating nucleation of the autophagosomal membrane. Membrane elongation is based on two essential steps: the assembly of Atg5-Atg12-Atg16 and the Atg5-Atg12-Atg16-mediated conjugation of LC3 I with phosphatidylethanolamine (PE). PE conjugated LC3 (i.e., LC3 II) stably associates with the autophagosomal vesicle, representing a widely used autophagosomal marker. Intracellular material is enclosed into autophagosomes during elongation and vesicle closure. Following closure, mature autophagosomes fuse with lysosomes, generating single-membrane autolysosomes. Autophagosomes can also fuse with endosomes to produce amphisomes, providing a point of convergence between the autophagic and endosomal pathways. Finally, cellular material is degraded in autolysosomes with the help of lysosomal enzymes and recycled, completing the cycle of autophagic flux[4,6].

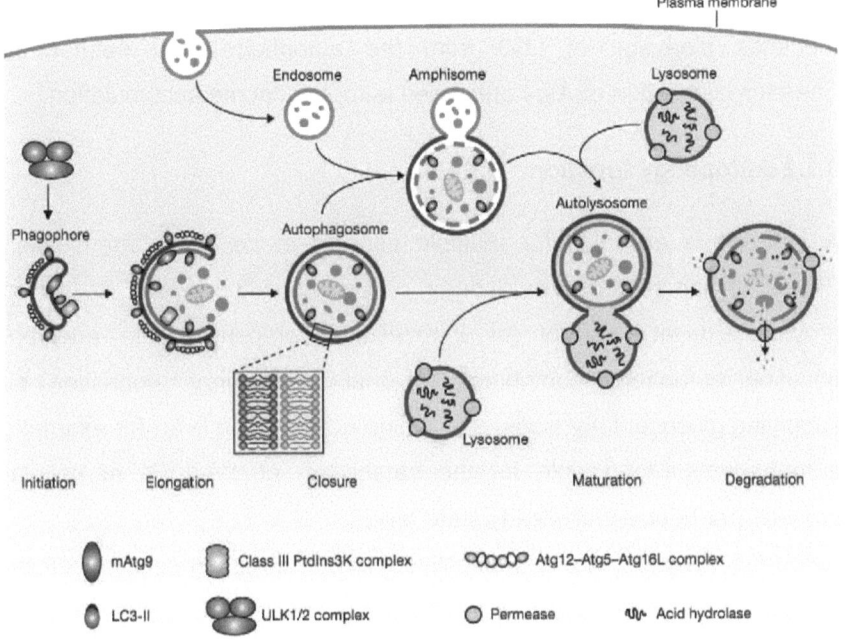

Figure 1: Schematic overview of autophagy (see text). The double membrane of autophagosomes is shown in detail. Adapted from Yang Z and Klionsky DJ[3] and published with permission.

Autophagy can be regulated at multiple points throughout the pathway[6]. Firstly, when nutrients are plentiful on a cellular level ULK complex can be inhibited by mTORC1. Starvation-mediated dissociation of mTORC1 activates ULK, initiating autophagy. Furthermore, Beclin-1 associates with multiple activators and inhibitors (e.g., Bif-1/UVRAG, Bcl-2/Bcl-xL). In addition, Atg5 can be cleaved and inactivated by calpains, which are cytosolic proteases that are dependent on high calcium concentrations. Atg5 is essential for LC3 I lipidation and autophagosome formation. Thus, reduction and/or absence of Atg5 blocks autophagosome formation. Finally, several proteins and signals can act on the level of

LC3. ROS, for example, can inhibit Atg4 proteolytic activity. Atg4 mediates cleavage of LC3 from the autophagosomal membrane. Therefore, inhibition of Atg4 enhances autophagosome accumulation.

3.1.2 Autophagy function

Autophagy is essential for multiple aspects of cellular homeostasis[5]. Baseline, non-selective autophagy occurs constitutively at low rates providing quality control for intracellular components. In addition, baseline autophagy contributes to anabolism/energy production by supplying glucose, fatty acids, and amino acids. In the liver, for example, autophagy is responsible for the catabolism of 1%-1.5% of cellular proteins per hour under steady state levels.

Autophagy can also act in a selective manner, targeting specific cellular components[5-8]. Among the targeted components are organelles such as peroxisomes, mitochondria, ER, ribosomes, and invading organisms (e.g., bacteria, viruses) as well as protein aggregates. Selective autophagy requires autophagic adaptor proteins. Adaptor proteins interact simultaneously with LC3 on nascent autophagosomes and the target substrate. Multiple adaptor proteins have been identified, such as p62, NDP52, and BNIP3/BNIP3L that are involved in different aspects of selective autophagy: p62 binds ubiquitinated proteins and protein aggregates, NDP52 sequesters invading pathogens, and both BNIP3/BNIP3L are important receptors for mitochondrial autophagy[8].

Autophagy induction can occur through a variety of stimuli[6]. Nutrient and energy stress are potent inducers of autophagy acting mainly via AMPK/mTORC1 signaling pathways. ER stress, initiated, for example, by accumulation of misfolded proteins and polyubiquitin aggregates, may positively regulate autophagic degradation. In addition, pathogen recognition receptors (e.g., toll-like receptors), which bind to invading microorganisms as well as products of necrotic cells and ROS, stimulate MAPK and NFκB-pathways, ultimately inducing autophagy. Moreover, mitochondrial damage, ROS-signaling and downstream effects, such as DNA-damage and p53 activation, activate autophagy. Among the latter, mitochondrial damage has a very important role since it induces a specialized form of autophagy called mitophagy, required for organelle removal and maintenance of energetic and oxidative homeostasis. Finally, hypoxia and anoxia may also cause autophagy via HIF, DJ-1, AMPK, or the unfolded protein response (UPR).

3.1.3 Autophagy and disease

As described above, autophagy is a cytoprotective mechanism enabling adaptation of cells to stressful conditions. Ultimately, autophagy maintains cellular energy balance, general homeostasis and function, allowing cells to survive multiple stressors[6]. Importantly, autophagy not only protects cells but also tissues and entire organisms from damage and various diseases. Disease associations have recently been established by studying tissue-specific knockouts of *Atg* genes, especially *Atg5* and *Atg7*. Whole-body knockouts of autophagy-genes (e.g., *Atg5*, *Atg7*) are not viable and lead to early postnatal lethality. An overview of various diseases associated with autophagy will be given in this section[5].

Neurons are terminally differentiated cells and cannot divide. Therefore, neurons critically depend on the housekeeping functions of autophagy. Indeed, knockout of autophagy in the central nervous system of mice causes neurologic deficits and loss of neuronal subtypes. Accumulation of ubiquitin and p62-positive protein aggregates is commonly observed upon autophagy deficiency. Aggregate formation, however, does not underlie reduced neuronal survival, since co-deletion of p62 abrogates aggregate formation without improving cellular survival[5]. Nevertheless, multiple neurodegenerative diseases are associated with autophagy[5] and stimulation of autophagy has been suggested as disease treatment[9]. Cardiac and skeletal muscle cells also depend on autophagy. Autophagy deficiency in cardiomyocytes leads to cardiac hypertrophy and dysfunction, owing to the accumulation of polyubiquitin aggregates. Damaged mitochondria were also observed after autophagy suppression during embryogenesis. In addition, autophagy is activated after pressure overload in the heart. Autophagy-deficient skeletal muscle cells exhibit similar morphological abnormalities, p62/polyubiquitin aggregates and deformed mitochondria, a condition resulting in muscle atrophy. Interestingly, autophagy has been associated with various neuromuscular disorders and myopathies supporting its importance in muscle homeostasis[5].

In the lung, defective autophagy has been associated with various pulmonary diseases (e.g., cystic fibrosis). Blockage of autophagy in bronchial epithelial cells results in p62-accumulation and Nrf2-activation (see below), indicating increased cytotoxic stress[5]. The function of autophagy in bone remains unknown. Nevertheless, an association with bone diseases has been established since *Sqstm1*-mutations (encoding p62) are detectable in Paget disease and immature autophagosomes accumulate in inclusion body myopathy associated with Paget disease and frontotemporal dementia[5].

Autophagy is also important in the gastrointestinal system. For example, intestinal Paneth cells rely on functional autophagy. Loss of autophagy results in secretory granule disorganization and is linked to Crohn's disease. Importantly, a single nucleotide polymorphism in *Atg16L1* has been associated with human Crohn's disease[5]. In the liver, loss of autophagy has been associated with hepatitis and hepatomas.

Accumulation of polyubiquitinated proteins and damaged mitochondria are direct consequences of autophagy deficiency and causative for the observed phenotype. Moreover, podocytes and renal tubules of the kidney exhibit high levels of autophagy. Tissue-specific autophagy-deficiency results in ubiquitinated protein aggregates, deformed organelles, and increased susceptibility to renal diseases[5].
Finally, recent studies have established an important role of autophagy in tumorigenesis. Interestingly, autophagy can function in both tumor initiation and tumor inhibition. For details see White E [10].

3.1.4 P62: more than an autophagic adaptor protein

p62 was originally identified as a binding partner for protein tyrosine kinase Lck[11]. Later on, p62 emerged as an autophagic adaptor protein as well as a prominent regulator of multiple intracellular signaling pathways[1,12].
Structurally, p62 possesses many protein-interaction domains, highlighting its scaffolding function (Figure 2). Firstly, p62 can interact with LC3 via an LC3-interacting region (i.e., LIR), with ubiquitinated proteins via an ubiquitin-associated (i.e., UBA) domain and with atypical protein kinase Cs (i.e., αPKC), including additional p62 molecules via a Phox and Bmep1 (i.e., PB1) domain. Consequently, p62 can target ubiquitinated proteins to autophagosomes and form multimers. Among the targets of p62 are ubiquitinated peroxisomes, mitochondria, protein aggregates, ribosomes, midbody rings, and viral/microbial proteins[1,12]. PB1 also mediates interaction with ERK1, blocking ERK1-signaling, a pathway that is especially important during adipogenesis[1]. Moreover, p62 can regulate NFκB-signaling. Binding to RIP, a component of TNF-signaling, or to TRAF6, in response to interleukin 1, nerve growth factor, or RANK ligand, activates pro-survival NFκB[1,12]. NFκB activation plays a

crucial role in osteoclastogenesis and Ras-induced carcinogenesis[1]. On the other hand, p62 can promote aggregation of ubiquitinated caspase-8, leading to enzyme activation and apoptosis induction[12]. Furthermore, p62 plays a role in nutrient sensing. In response to amino acid starvation, p62 was shown to mediate docking of mTORC1 on lysosomes, which is crucial for mTORC1 activation[13].

Nrf2-dependent expression of antioxidant and detoxifying genes is another pathway regulated by p62. p62 inhibits proteasome-mediated degradation of Nrf2 by blocking interaction of Nrf2 with Keap1, the E3-ubiquitin ligase for Nrf2[1,12]. Nrf2 also induces *Sqstm1* transcription pointing to a positive feedback loop[12].

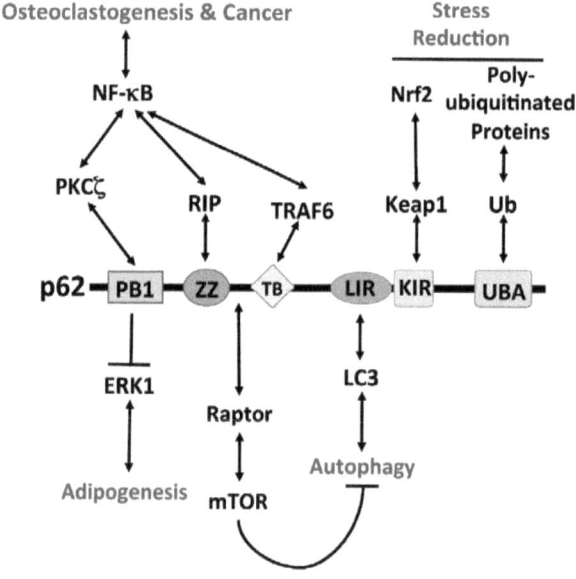

Figure 2: p62 domains, interacting partners and function[1]. Published with permission.

p62 protein levels are regulated by autophagy[12]. Therefore, the immediate effect of autophagy defects is p62 accumulation. Since p62 is able to oligomerize, accumulation of p62 upon autophagy defects results in aggregate and, ultimately, inclusion body formation[12,14]. Aggregates have been described in autophagy-deficient brain, liver, kidney, lung, and muscle[5]. In the liver p62-aggregates seem to be causative for the autophagy-deficient phenotype, since simultaneous knockout of p62 abolishes aggregates and ameliorates liver injury[5].

Autophagy deficiency and p62-accumulation also perturb p62-associated signaling pathways. Importantly, constitutive NFκB-activation occurring with increased p62 protein levels supports tumorigenesis, as shown for lung[15] and pancreas[16]. On the other hand, excess p62 during states of autophagy defects, may also cause inhibition of canonical NFκB signaling, leading to non-canonical NFκB-activation and enhanced liver tumorigenesis[17]. Finally, autophagy defects influence Nrf2-signaling. Importantly, p62/Keap1 aggregates are detectable in human hepatocellular carcinoma along with Nrf2-target gene expression[18]. In addition, mutations in *NFE2L2/KEAP1* have been observed in human cancers. These mutations along with other Nrf2-pathway modifications result in continuous Nrf2-activation and resistance to chemotherapy[12]. Moreover, Nrf2-activation might be causative for aggregation of ubiquitinated proteins upon autophagy deficiency, since ubiquitin aggregates disappear in liver and brain after simultaneous deletion of either *Sqstm1* or *Nfe2l2*[19]. Interestingly, Nrf2 is able to influence transcription of ubiquitin-associated genes, further highlighting the importance of Nrf2 in influencing cellular homeostasis[19].

Functional autophagy therefore is not only important for the maintenance of cellular homeostasis but also for selective degradation of adaptor molecules such as p62. Removal of p62 aggregates alleviates persistent activation or inhibition of signaling pathways, restoring normal signaling and cellular function.

3.2 Pancreas

3.2.1 Morphology and function

The pancreas is an abdominal organ and is located in close proximity to the duodenum, spleen, and the common bile duct[20]. The pancreas exerts two main functions: aiding intestinal nutrient digestion and secreting hormones (e.g., insulin, glucagon, amylin, somatostatin, and pancreatic polypeptide) into the circulation. Thus, the pancreas can be separated into exocrine and endocrine portions, containing acinar tissue with a duct system (approximately 85% of pancreatic mass) and islets of Langerhans, respectively. Both tissue types are interspersed and interact through direct blood flow from islets to acinar cells, enabling transfer of hormones to exocrine cells[20].
Islets of Langerhans consist of a variety of specialized cells, named alpha, beta, delta, PP, and epsilon cells all organized into a cluster. Every cell type produces distinct hormones secreted directly into the blood flow. Exocrine pancreatic tissue consists of multiple acini, each with separate draining ductules, which connect to the duodenum via interlobular ducts and the main pancreatic ductal system. Single acini are made of acinar cells. Acinar cells produce, store, and secrete multiple digestive enzymes (including amylase, lipase, and others), as well as inactive preforms of digestive enzymes (i.e., zymogens, such as trypsinogen, chymotrypsinogen, proelastase, and others), and other factors that are essential for digestive and absorptive functions (e.g., bicarbonate, colipase, and others). Epithelial cells of the ductular system secrete bicarbonate required for neutralization of gastric acid and optimal

pancreatic enzyme function. Centroacinar cells are localized at the junction of acinus and ductule, produce bicarbonate, and likely serve as progenitor cells for multiple pancreatic cells.

Acinar cells exhibit the highest rate of protein synthesis among all mammalian cell types. Accordingly, acinar cells require a highly developed ER, extensive protein folding machinery, organelles for enzyme storage, and multiple mitochondria to satisfy the energy needs required for protein synthesis. Along this route of protein synthesis and secretion, multiple genetic and environmental challenges may occur, leading e.g., to ER stress. Thus, pancreatic acinar cells need to be able to adapt to stressors and changing demands; failure to adapt will disturb pancreatic function and result in disease conditions described below.

3.2.2 Pancreatic Pathology

Digestive enzymes and zymogens are stored in zymogen granules[20]. The acidic milieu within zymogen granules and the co-localization with a trypsin inhibitor (i.e., PSTI or SPINK) prevent autocatalytic activation of trypsinogen to trypsin. Controlled activation occurs in the duodenum, where the enzyme enterokinase cleaves trypsinogen activation peptide (TAP) from trypsinogen leaving trypsin; trypsin then activates the remaining zymogens, enabling digestion of macromolecular nutrients. Premature activation of zymogens leads to pancreatic autodigestion, tissue damage, and pancreatic inflammation (i.e., pancreatitis).

Acute pancreatic injury resulting in intra-acinar zymogen activation, decreased pancreatic enzyme secretion, inflammation, and cell death constitute acute pancreatitis (AP)[2]. The annual incidence of AP in humans ranges from 13 to 45/100.000 persons[21]. AP is associated with multiple risk factors such as increasing age, alcohol, smoking, visceral obesity, diabetes mellitus, gallstones, hypertriglyceridemia, autoimmune disease, and certain genetic mutations[21]. In most cases, AP is self-limiting and mild, characterized by abdominal pain, pancreatic necrosis, and increased amylase and lipase activities in serum or plasma[22]. However, 20% of patients develop severe disease with systemic complications including multiple organ failure and death[22]. Moreover, recurrent episodes of AP may also occur (20-30% of patients)[21]. Mortality is low, but increases when necrotic regions within the pancreas occur, which are frequently associated with pancreatic infections[22].

Approximately 10% of human patients with AP develop chronic pancreatitis (CP)[21]. The annual incidence of CP ranges from 5 to 12/100.000 persons[21]. Risk factors for CP include alcohol and smoking; CP is also more common among males[21]. Clinically, CP is associated with chronic inflammation, fibrosis, pancreatic atrophy, and loss of acinar and islet cell function, potentially leading to exocrine and endocrine insufficiency, a process that can take many years[23]. Survival time of CP-patients is lower than the general population, but usual causes of mortality are non-pancreatic in origin[21]. Management of patients with CP greatly depends on accurate diagnosis, determination of etiology, and constant monitoring since clinical manifestations differ between patients and may include multiple complications[23].

Figure 3 illustrates potential associations between acute and chronic pancreatitis. Recently, autophagy has been shown to influence multiple steps in pancreatic disease progression. The following section describes some of these steps.

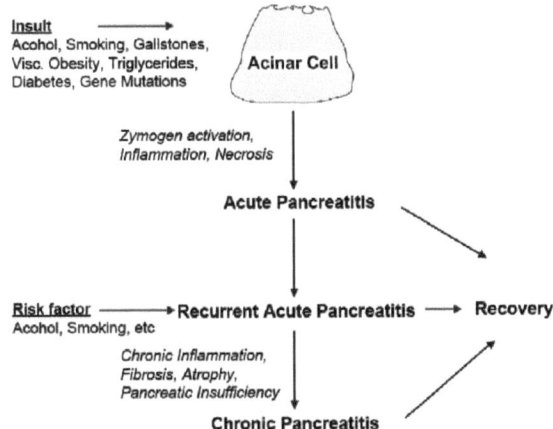

Figure 3: Relationship between acute and chronic pancreatitis[2].

3.3 Pancreas and autophagy

Past studies have associated autophagy with endocrine and exocrine pancreatic physiology. In endocrine β-cells, basal autophagy prevents accumulation of ubiquitinated proteins, p62, deformed mitochondria, and ER, maintaining β-cell function and normal insulin production[5]. Moreover, free fatty acids induce autophagy in β-cells initiating an adaptive response important during the presence of insulin resistance[5].

In the exocrine pancreas, baseline and starvation-induced autophagy levels are higher compared to those of other organs[24]. Pancreatic acinar cells are known for their high rate of protein synthesis. Thus, autophagy has been hypothesized as a mechanism for removing excessive and damaged proteins and adjusting zymogen granule number to the needs of the organism[24]. So far however, this has not been definitively established[24].

A hallmark feature of experimental and human pancreatitis is acinar cell vacuolization[24]. Recently it has been suggested that these vacuoles are predominantly autolysosomes containing undegraded material[24,25]. Importantly, accumulation of vacuoles is accompanied by increased LC3II and p62 levels along with a decreased rate of protein degradation, suggesting compromised autophagic flux[24]. Mechanistically, pancreatitis does not inhibit fusion of autophagosomes with lysosomes, neither does it block autophagosome formation[24]. Pancreatitis even appears to further stimulate autophagosome formation[24]. Indeed, impaired lysosomal function has been shown to block autophagic flux during pancreatitis due to defective lysosomal enzyme activity and reduced expression of lysosomal membrane protein[24]. In addition, dysfunctional lysosomes mediate pathological trypsin activation by causing an imbalance between cathepsin L and cathepsin B levels resulting in reduced cathepsin L levels. Cathepsin L is involved in trypsinogen degradation, whereas cathepsin B activates trypsinogen; thus trypsin accumulates in acinar cells during pancreatitis[2].

Furthermore, autophagy has been associated with CP. In particular, chronic inflammation and fibrosis, which are central hallmarks of CP, appear to be regulated by autophagy[2,24]. Increased p62-levels upon autophagy deficiency may activate NFκB-signaling, thus initiating an inflammatory response[2]. Furthermore, lack of mitochondrial autophagy results in accumulation of damaged mitochondria, ROS-production, and inflammasome activation[2]. Inflammasomes persist in autophagy-deficient cells, since autophagy regulates inflammasome elimination[2]. Loss of removal of apoptotic material inside acinar cells induces necrosis and release of damage-associated molecular pattern molecules, constituting another link with chronic inflammation[2]. Moreover, autophagy has been shown to regulate fibrosis in the liver[24,26], and influence pancreatic stellate cell survival[27], the main fibrogenic cell type of the pancreas. Taken together, autophagic degradation is required for maintenance of normal pancreatic physiology and function. Importantly, defects in autophagy are associated with common pancreatic diseases, making pancreatic autophagy an important field of study for future investigations on pancreatic function and pathology.

3.4 Aim

The central aim of the present study was to elucidate the function of autophagy in pancreatic physiology and disease by using an *in vivo* model of autophagy deficiency. Pancreas-specific *Atg5*-knockout mice were generated and characterized at various time-points after birth. Transcriptomics and metabolomics were performed to assess changes in pancreatic physiology caused by autophagy deficiency. Stress-resistance was analyzed in experimental models of pancreatitis. Specific dietary formulations were applied to scrutinize the influence of dietary composition on pancreatic pathology. Moreover, the importance of p53 and p62 in Atg5-dependent autophagy was analyzed by using pancreas-specific *Trp53/Atg5* and *Sqstm1/Atg5* double deficient mice.

4 MATERIALS AND METHODS

4.1 Mice

4.1.1 Mouse models

- $Atg5^{flox/flox}$ [28]: Exon 3 of $Atg5$ was flanked by two loxP sites.
- $Sqstm1^{flox/flox}$ [29]: Exon 1 of $Sqstm1$ was flanked by two loxP sites.
- $Trp53^{flox/flox}$ [30]: loxP sites were placed in intron 1 and 10 of $Trp53$.
- $Ptf1a$-cre^{ex1} [31]: Part of exon 1 (ex1) in the $Ptf1a$ locus was replaced with the Cre recombinase.
- $Elastase$-$CreER^{TM}$ [32]: An enhancer of the Elastase gene was fused to a minimal hsp68 promoter and placed upstream of a $CreER^{TM}$ coding sequence. $ElaCre;A5^{F/F}$ mice were used for conditional knockout of $Atg5$ in adult acinar cells.
- $Gt(ROSA)26Sor^{tm4(ACTB-tdTomato,-EGFP)Luo/J}$ (007576 Jackson Laboratory[33]): The construct consisted of a CMV enhancer and β-actin core promoter (pCA) regulating transcription of loxP flanked membrane-targeted tandem dimer $Tomato$. The resulting protein was therefore localized to cellular membranes. Membrane-targeted enhanced green fluorescent protein was produced after Cre-mediated excision of $Tomato$.
- GFP-$LC3$ transgenic mice[34]: Rat $LC3$ was fused to $EGFP$ at the N-terminus. Thus, GFP-$LC3$ transgenic mice expressed LC3 coupled to EGFP. Formation of autophagosomes led to increased detection of GFP-LC3 puncta, enabling analysis of autophagy induction[34]. Background fluorescence was seen under conditions without autophagy stimulation.

Mouse strain combinations included:

$Atg5^{flox/flox}$; $Ptf1a$-cre^{ex1} (termed A5), $Atg5^{flox/flox}$ (termed $A5^{F/F}$, used as control wherever indicated) and $Atg5^{flox/+}$;$Ptf1a$-cre^{ex1} (termed $A5^{F/-}$, used as control wherever indicated), $Atg5^{flox/flox}$; $Sqstm1^{flox/flox}$; $Ptf1a$-cre^{ex1} (termed A5;p62), $Sqstm1^{flox/flox}$; $Ptf1a$-cre^{ex1} (termed p62), $Atg5^{flox/flox}$; $Trp53^{flox/flox}$; $Ptf1a$-cre^{ex1} (termed A5;p53), $Atg5^{flox/flox}$; $Gt(ROSA)26Sor^{tm4(ACTB-tdTomato,-EGFP)Luo/J}$ combined with $Ptf1a$-cre^{ex1} (termed Tom-GFP A5) or $Elastase$-$CreER^{TM}$ (termed Tom-GFP ElaCre;A5), $Atg5^{flox/flox}$; $Elastase$-$CreER^{TM}$ (termed ElaCre;A5)

For all the experiments in this study, mice were housed under specific pathogen-free conditions with free access to food and water. The Regierung von Oberbayern reviewed and approved all animal procedures.

4.1.2 Acute pancreatitis

Sex-matched, 8 week old littermates (8-12 week-old) had food withheld for 12-18 hours. Water was provided ad libitum. Mice received eight hourly, intraperitoneal (i.p.) injections of 50 µg/kg body weight cerulein (5 µg/ml, Sigma, Munich, Germany) diluted in 0.9% saline according to the scheme in Figure 22. Mice were sacrificed 0h, 24h or 4 days after the first injection of cerulein. Serum was obtained at 0h and 4h after the first injection of cerulein.

For analysis of GFP-LC3 puncta formation, mice were treated with cerulein for 1 day as described above and sacrificed 4 or 8 h after the first injection. Alternatively, mice were treated for 3 consecutive days with cerulein as described above and sacrificed thereafter.

4.1.3 Dietary modifications

A palm oil enriched diet (S5745-E712, ssniff, Soest, Germany) or a standard murine diet (1310, Altromin, Lage, Germany) was given to male $A5$ and $A5^{F/F}$ mice according to the scheme in Figure 24A. Detailed comparison between diets can be seen in Table 12. Alternatively, drinking water was supplemented with 40 mM N-acetylcysteine (Sigma), according to the scheme in Figure 24A. Dietary modifications started at 4 weeks of age and ended at 18 weeks of age. Serum glucose and IPGTT were analyzed prior to sacrifice. After sacrifice, mice were weighed and the pancreas was examined. Experiments were repeated three times, independent of each other.

4.1.4 Induction of *ElastaseCre* expression

Cre-Recombinase expression was induced in 4-week old *ElaCre;A5* or $A5^{F/F}$ mice by i.p. injection of 1 mg/15 g body weight tamoxifen (T5648, Sigma) for three consecutive days according to the scheme in Figure 10A. Mice were sacrificed at 9 or 18 weeks of age. Acute pancreatitis was induced in *ElaCre;A5* and $A5^{F/F}$ mice as described above and according to the scheme in Figure 11.

4.1.5 Glucose Measurement and Intraperitoneal Glucose Tolerance Test (IPGTT)

Random serum glucose concentration was measured in 18-week old male and female $A5$ and $A5^{F/F}$ mice fed SD or male $A5$ and $A5^{F/F}$ mice fed POD. Mice were given free access to food and water. A drop of blood was obtained from the tail vein and directly analyzed with the Accu-Chek Inform II system (Roche, Mannheim, Germany).

For IPGTT, food was withheld for 12-18 h from 18-week old male, POD-fed $A5$ and $A5^{F/F}$ mice. Glucose (2 g/kg body weight) was i.p. injected and serum glucose was measured from the tail vein prior to injection (0 min), as well as 15, 30, 60, 90, and 120 min after injection. Food was returned to mice after last measurement.

4.2 DNA/RNA studies

4.2.1 Mouse genotyping

Genotyping of mice was performed by DNA extraction from the tail tip of mice. Tail tips were obtained from mice at 4 weeks of age (standard genotyping) or after sacrifice (post-genotyping) to verify genotype. Tails were lysed in Tail Lysis Buffer (100mM TRIS/HCl (Sigma) pH 8.5; 200mM NaCl (Sigma); 5mM EDTA (Sigma) pH 8.0; 0.2% SDS (Sigma); 5% Proteinase K (Roche)) for 2-12 hours at 60°C. During and after the incubation, samples were thoroughly mixed and incubated for 10 minutes at 95°C to inactivate the proteinase K. To dilute the DNA, dH2O (900μl) was added. Genotyping PCR was performed with 3-5 μl of DNA using the RedTaq Ready Mix (Sigma). A standard PCR protocol was applied (Table 1). All primers (Table 2) were used at a final concentration of 10 pM. Mice were genotyped with the assistance of Karen Dlubatz and Chantal Geisert.

Table 1: Genotyping PCR standard protocol.

Step	Temperature	Time	Cycle number
Pre-incubation	95°C	5 min	1x
Amplification	95°C	30 sec	35x
	60°C	30sec	
	72°C	60 sec	
Cooling	4°C	∞	1x

Table 2: Genotyping primer sequences and product sizes.

Name	Primer forward (5´-3´)	Primer reverse (5´-3´)	Product (bp)
Atg5 wildtype	GAATATGAAGGCAC ACCCCTGAAATG	GTACTGCATAATGGTTT AACTCTTGC	350
Atg5$^{F/F}$	ACAACGTCGAGCAC AGCTGCGCAAGG	GTACTGCATAATGGTTT AACTCTTGC	700
Sqstm1	GGCAATGGCTGGTC TACTTT	GGACTGAGCCTCTGAG CAAC	Wildtype: 449 Mutated: 547
Trp53	CACAAAAACAGGTTA AACCCAG	AGCACATAGGAGGCAG AGAC	Wildtype: 280 Mutated: 350
GFP-LC3	TCCTGCTGGAGTTC GTGACCG	TTGCGAATTCTCAGCC GTCTTCATCTCTCTCGC	400
Tomato wildtype	CTCTGCTGCCTCCT GGCTTCT	CGAGGCGGATCACAAG CAATA	330
Tomato$^{F/F}$	CTCTGCTGCCTCCT GGCTTCT	TCAATGGGCGGGGT CGTT	250
Cre	ACCAGCCAGCTATC AACTCG	TTACATTGGTCCAGCC ACC	Wildtype: 350 Mutated: 200
	CTAGGCCACAGAAT TGAAAGATCT	GTAGGTGGAAATTCTA GCATCATCC	
CreRT^{TM}	GAT TTA CGG CGC TAA GGA TGA CT	AGG GTG CTG GAC AGA AAT GTG TA	800

4.2.2 RNA extraction

For RNA extraction, mice were sacrificed and samples of the pancreas were immediately removed, homogenized in RLT lysis buffer (1015762 Qiagen, Hilden, Germany) supplemented with 1% β-mercaptoethanol (M6250 Sigma) and snap frozen. Subsequently, RNA was extracted using the RNeasy Mini Kit (74104 Qiagen). NanoDrop 2000 spectrophotometer (Peqlab, Erlangen, Germany) was used to determine RNA concentration and RNA purity through the absorbance ratios at 260 nm/280 nm and 260 nm/230 nm.

4.2.3 cDNA synthesis

SuperScript II Reverse Transcriptase (18064-014 Invitrogen, Darmstadt Germany) along with 1-5 µg RNA was used for complementary DNA (cDNA) synthesis. The reaction mix included oligo(dt)$_{12-18}$ primer. cDNA obtained from the reaction was quantified and concentration set to 20 ng/µl.

4.2.4 Quantitative real time PCR analysis

Quantitative RT-PCR was performed on a LightCycler 480 (Roche) using the LightCycler 480 Sybr Green Master Mix 1 (Roche). Reaction conditions can be seen in table 3. 100 ng cDNA were used as a template. Target mRNA expression was normalized to endogenous *Cyclophilin* and quantified by the delta-delta CT method ($2^{DeltaCT(Cyclophilin) - DeltaCT(target\ gene)}$). Melting curves were evaluated to verify primer specificity. Primers are listed in table 4.

Table 3: qRT-PCR program.

Step	Temperature	Time	Cycle number
Pre-incubation	95°C	10 min	1x
Amplification	95°C	10 sec	45x
	60°C	20 sec	
	72°C	10 sec	
Melting	95°C	1 min	
	55°C	1 sec	
	98°C	Continuous 0.11°C/sec	5 acquisitions/sec
Cooling	37°C	5 min	1x

Table 4: qRT-PCR primer sequences and product sizes.

Name	Primer forward (5´-3´)	Primer reverse (5´-3´)	Product (bp)
Amylase	TGGTCAATGGTCAGCCTTTTTC	CACAGTATGTGCCAGCAGGAAG	153
Elastase	GCCTGCTGGTTGTGGACTAT	GTAGTTGCAGCCCAGAGAGG	206
Bhlha15 (Mist1)	TGACCGCCACCATACTTACTA	GCTGGTATAATTTAGGGCCTGG	87
Hnf1b	CACCAAGCCGGTTTTCCATAC	GGAGTGTCATAGTCGTCGCC	96
Nrf1	TCTCACCCTCCAAACCCAAC	CCCGACCTGTGGAATACTTG	255
Nfe2l2	TTCTTTCAGCAGCATCCTCTCCAC	ACAGCCTTCAATAGTCCCGTCCAG	199
Nqo1	CACGGGGACATGAACGTCAT	GGAGTGTGGCCAATGCTGTA	107
Hmox1	CACGCATATACCCGCTACCT	CCAGAGTGTTCATTCGAGCA	175
Gclc	ATGACTGTTGCCAGGTGGATGAGA	ACACGCCATCCTAAACAGCGATCA	254

Sqstm1	TGTGGAACATGGAGGGAAGAG	TGTGCCTGTGCTGGAACTTTC	67
Atf3	CGAAGACTGGAGCAAAATGATG	CAGGTTAGCAAAATCCTCAAATAC	127
Hspa5	ACTTGGGGACCACCTATTCCT	ATCGCCAATCAGACGCTCC	134
Ddit3	CTGGAAGCCTGGTATGAGGAT	CAGGGTCAAGAGTAGTGAAGGT	121
Ppp1r15a	GCCTGCAAGGGGCTGATAAG	TTTGTATCCCGGAGCTATGGA	173
Edem1	GCAATGAAGGAGAAGGAGACCC	TAGAAGGCGTGTAGGCAGATGG	157
Dnajc3	TTTACTGCCGCAAGACTACAG	CTGGGGTTAGATTTGAGCACTT	101
P4hb	CAAGATCAAGCCCCACCTGAT	AGTTCGCCCCAACCAGTACTT	83
Xbp1	ACACGCTTGGGAATGGACAC	CCATGGGAAGATGTTCTGGG	-Xbp1u 171 -Xbp1s 145
Trp53	AGATCCGCGGGCGTAAAC	TCTGTAGCATGGGCATCCTTT	79
Cdkn1a	CCTGGTGATGTCCGACCTG	CCATGAGCGCATCGCAATC	103
Bax	AGACAGGGGCCTTTTTGCTAC	AATTCGCCGGAGACACTCG	137
Bak1	CAGCTTGCTCTCATCGGAGAT	GGTGAAGAGTTCGTAGGCATTC	108
Cyclophilin A	ATGGTCAACCCCACCGTGT	TTCTGCTGTCTTTGGAACTTTGTC	102

4.2.5 Detection of unspliced and spliced *Xbp1*

For detection of *Xbp1* whole pancreatic cDNA was subjected to PCR with a primer set detecting both unspliced (171 bp) and spliced (145 bp) *Xbp1* (Table 4). PCR conditions can be seen in Table 5. PCR products were separated by agarose gel electrophoresis. *Cyclophilin* was used as control.

Table 5: PCR conditions for detection of unspliced and spliced *Xbp1*.

Step	Temperature	Time	Cycle number
Pre-incubation	94°C	4 min	1x
Amplification	94°C	10 sec	35x
	65°C	30 sec	
	72°C	30 sec	
Extension	72°C	10 min	1x
Cooling	4°C	∞	1x

4.2.6 Agarose gel electrophoresis

For agarose gel electrophoresis, agarose (Biozym, Hess. Oldendorf) was dissolved by heating in 1xTAE-Buffer (0.4 M Tris, 0.2 M acetic glacial acid, 0.01 M EDTA x NA_2 x $2H_2O$) at a concentration from 1 to 3% (w/v), dependent on PCR-product size. After cooling down to approximately 50°C, ethidium bromide (Sigma) was added to the agarose solution at a final concentration of 0.5 µg/ml. The agarose solution was poured into an electrophoresis chamber and allowed to polymerize. PCR-products diluted in loading buffer (Peqlab) along with a DNA-ladder (Peqlab, 1 kb) were run horizontally at 100 V. Documentation was performed by UV-light (EX/EM 312/516-518 nm, GelDoc™XR system)

4.2.7 Microarray analysis

RNA isolation and Affymetrix GeneChip (*Mus musculus*) Mouse Gene 1.0 ST Array was conducted by Kompetenzzentrum Fluoreszente Bioanalytik (KFB) Regensburg. Gene set enrichment analysis software (GSEA) provided by the Broad Institute was utilized to analyze the microarray data. For a selected number of genes (i.e., those depicted in

Figure 15), the normalized log2 Signal Values obtained from the microarray analysis were used to calculate averages ± standard deviations. Two-sided Student's t-test was used to compare *A5* and *A5*$^{F/F}$ mice.

4.2.8 *Atg5* exon sequencing in humans with CP

This portion of the study was reviewed and approved by the medical ethical review committee of the TUM. All enrolled individuals had given written informed consent prior to enrolment. The diagnosis of CP was based on two or more of the following criteria: presence of a typical history of recurrent pancreatitis, pancreatic calcifications and/or pancreatic ductal irregularities revealed by endoscopic retrograde pancreatography (ERCP) or by magnetic resonance imaging of the pancreas, and/or consistent sonographic findings. Hereditary CP was diagnosed when one first-degree relative or two or more second-degree relatives suffered from recurrent AP or CP without any apparent precipitating factor. Affected individuals were classified as having idiopathic CP when precipitating factors, such as alcohol abuse, trauma, medication, infection, metabolic disorders, or a positive family history were absent. The study included 267 unrelated patients with idiopathic/hereditary CP (159 female and 108 male patients; median age 12 years, mean age 14.8 years, range 0-70 years) as well as 241 healthy blood donors as controls (119 female, 122 male; median age 22 years, mean age 24.4 years, range 18-61 years).

For *ATG5* exon sequence analysis, DNA was extracted from peripheral blood leukocytes. All 7 coding exons and the exon-intron boundaries of *ATG5* were analyzed by uni-directional DNA sequencing. Primers (Table 6) were complementary to intronic sequences flanking *ATG5* coding exons based on the published nucleotide sequence (ensemble:

ENSG00000057663). Oligonucleotides were synthesized by TIB MOLBIOL, Berlin, Germany. PCR was performed using 0.75 U AmpliTaq Gold polymerase (Thermo Fisher Scientific, Schwerte, Germany), 400 µmol/l deoxynucleoside triphosphates, and 0.1 µmol/l primers in a total volume of 25 µl. Cycle conditions were as follows: initial denaturation for 12 min at 95°C; 48 cycles of 20 s denaturation at 95°C, 40 s annealing at 60°C, 90 s primer extension at 72°C; and a final extension step for 2 min at 72°C. PCR products were digested with Antarctic phosphatase (New England Biolabs, Frankfurt am Main, Germany) and exonuclease I (New England Biolabs). Cycle sequencing was performed using internal sequencing primers and BigDye terminator mix (Thermo Fisher Scientific) with an annealing temperature of 60°C. The reaction products were purified by ethanol precipitation and loaded onto an ABI 3730 fluorescence sequencer (Thermo Fisher Scientific).

DNA mutation numbering was based on the cDNA sequence (GenBank: NM_004849.2) that uses the A of the ATG start codon as nucleotide +1. The mutations were described according to the nomenclature recommended by the Human Genome Variation Society (http://www.hgvs.org/mutnomen).

Statistical analysis was carried out using a Fisher's exact test. P-values less than 0.05 were considered statistically significant. A commercial software package (SPSS software version 11.0 for Windows, Chicago, USA) was used to perform the statistical analyses. Data acquisition and analysis was done by Claudia Pilsak and Heiko Witt.

Table 6: Primer sequences used for PCR amplification and sequencing of *ATG5* coding regions.

Exon	PCR forward	PCR reverse	DNA sequencing
2	GCAGTAGACTCTTCTGGGCTTG	CATCATGACAACATGCTGACAGTGG	GAAGTGGATAATCTTTATGGCATGG
3	GATTTGTGTTGATCATTCTGGGC	CCATGCATCCAAACAGAAGGCAG	AAGCAGTAGACTTTGTGTGGG
4	GAGGTTTCTATGGGAATGGAGTGG	GCTTAGCAACTAAAACAGTGTCAGG	GATCATACTAGCCTAGGCACG
5	GTGTGAGGGCTCCATTCCAC	CAAATCTGGGCACAGAGGCTAC	GGGTTATTTCAGTGCTAAGAGATAG
6	GCGAATATCTAGGGAGAGGATGC	CTTGATTGCCACTGAAAGACACAG	GTCCTTTCAGAAACTTCTAGAGG
7	GCTAACACCGTATCAAAAGGCACC	CCAGTCGAGTCATCATTTTGTTAGTC	CGTATCAAAAGGCACCTAATGCC
8	TGCCACTACAGTTTCATTAACGTC	CCTGTCTGGCTTGCAGCAGC	CTGTTTTGGGTGATACATACTGC

4.3 Histology

4.3.1 Tissue sections

Paraffin sections

Mouse tissue samples were fixed in 4% PFA (Merck, Darmstadt, Germany)/PBS for 12-18 h, dehydrated and embedded in paraffin. A microtome (HM 355 S, MICROM, Walldorf, Germany) was used to cut 3.0-5.0 µm thick sections. Sections were mounted on adhesive-coated slides (SuperFrost® Plus, Menzel, Braunschweig, Germany) and air-dried at approximately 25°C for 12-18 h. Sections were kept at 25°C until further analysis.

Cryo-sections

Pancreatic tissue was snap frozen in freezing medium (Tissue-Tek O.C.T. Compound, Weckert Labortechnik, Kitzingen, Germany) and stored at -80°C. A cryotome (Cryo-Star HM 560 MV, MICROM) was used to cut 6-10 μm thick sections. Sections were mounted on adhesive-coated slides (SuperFrost® Plus, Menzel) and kept at -20°C until further analysis.

4.3.2 Haematoxylin and eosin (H&E) staining

For H&E staining, paraffin-embedded tissue sections were deparaffinized in xylol (Merck) for 2 x 5 minutes followed by rehydration in ethanol (100%, 96%, 70%; 3 minutes each) and water (2 x 3 minutes). The slides were incubated in haematoxylin solution (Merck Millipore, Billerica, MA) for 5 minutes, washed with running tap water for 10 minutes and incubated in eosin solution (Merck) for 3.5 minutes. Dehydration was performed with 96% Ethanol and Isopropanol for 25 sec each and xylol for 2 x 3 minutes. Slides were subsequently covered with mounting medium (pertex, Medite GmbH) and coverslips (Merck). Axiostar Plus (Carl Zeiss, Göttingen, Germany) was used for histological analysis.

4.3.3 Immunohistochemistry

For immunohistochemistry, slides were de-waxed and rehydrated as described under 4.3.2. Antigen retrieval was done by shortly boiling the slides in 0.01 M citrate buffer (pH 6.0) followed by sub-boiling for 10 minutes. Slides were allowed to cool down at approximately 25°C for 20 minutes in citrate buffer and washed 2 x 5 minutes with water. Endogenous peroxidase was blocked with 3% hydrogen peroxide for 15 min at approximately 25°C in the dark and slides were washed 2 x 5 minutes with wash buffer (TBS, TBS-T, PBS or PBS-T (Table 7) depending on the primary antibody). Nonspecific binding was blocked with blocking solution (5% rabbit or 5% goat serum, according to the secondary antibody, in wash buffer) for 1 h at approximately 25°C. Slides were then incubated with the primary antibody diluted in blocking solution (or wherever indicated in SignalStain antibody diluent, 8112 Cell Signaling Technology, Danvers, MA) for 12-18 h at 4°C. Primary antibodies used include: anti-BrdU (1/250; MCA2060 AbD Serotec, Puchheim, Germany), anti-cleaved caspase 3 (1/100 in SignalStain antibody diluent; 9661 Cell Signaling Technology), anti-Periostin (1/300; AP08724AF-N Acris, Herford, Germany), anti-F4/80 (1/100; MF-48,000 Invitrogen), anti-p62 (1/100; GP62-C Progen, Heidelberg, Germany), anti-Nqo1 (1/100; ab28947 abcam, Cambridge, UK), anti-p53 (1/500; NCL-p53-CM5p Novocastra, Wetzlar, Germany), anti-SOX9 (1/2,000 in SignalStain antibody diluent; 8112 Cell Signaling Technology), anti-HNF1β (1/500 in SignalStain antibody diluent; sc-22840 Santa Cruz, Heidelberg, Germany), anti-insulin (1/100; A0564 Dako, Hamburg, Germany), anti-γH2Ax (1/200; 05-636 Merck Millipore), anti-phosho-p38 (1/100; 4631 Cell Signaling Technology), anti-phospho-c-Jun (1/50; 9164 Cell Signaling Technology), anti-phospho-ERK (1/100; 4376 Cell Signaling Technology), and anti-phosphoSer276-p65 (1/50; 3037 Cell Signaling Technology). After incubation, slides were washed 3 x 5 minutes with wash buffer. Secondary antibodies including biotinylated anti-rabbit in goat (BA 1000 Vector Laboratories, Lörrach, Germany), anti-mouse in goat (BA 9200 Vector Laboratories), anti-rat in rabbit (BA 4000 Vector Laboratories) and horseradish peroxidase conjugated anti-guinea pig in goat (A7289 Sigma) were applied for 1 h at approximately 25°C with a concentration of 1/300-1/500 in blocking solution. Finally, slides were washed and signal detection was performed with avidin-biotin peroxidase complex for biotinylated secondary antibodies (Vector Laboratories) and DAB reagent (Vector Laboratories) according to the manufacturer's directions. In the case of horseradish peroxidase conjugated secondary antibodies, avidin-biotin peroxidase complex was not applied. Haematoxylin was used as a counterstain and slides were subsequently dehydrated and mounted as described (4.3.2).

Table 7: Buffers used for washing.

Name	Components	pH
TBS	20 mM Tris, 137 mM NaCl	7.6
TBS-T	TBS-buffer, 0.1% (v/v) Tween-20	7.6
PBS	137 mM NaCl, 2.7 mM KCl, 10 mM Na_2HPO_4, 10 mM KH_2PO_4	7.4
PBS-T	PBS-buffer, 0.1% (v/v) Tween-20	7.4

4.3.4 Co-immunofluorescence

Paraffin-embedded pancreatic tissue sections were de-waxed, rehydrated, and heated for antigen retrieval as described (4.3.3). Nonspecific binding was blocked with blocking solution (5% goat or 5% rabbit serum, according to the secondary antibody, in wash buffer (table 7)) for 1 h at approximately 25°C and incubated over two consecutive nights at 4°C with the first and second primary antibody, respectively. Primary antibodies were diluted in blocking solution (or wherever indicated in SignalStain antibody diluent 8112 Cell Signaling Technology) and included: anti-amylase (1/300; A8273 Sigma), anti-CK19 (1/200; TROMA III Developmental Studies Hybridoma Bank), anti-SOX9 (1/2,000 in SignalStain antibody diluent; 8112 Cell Signaling Technology), anti-Hes1 (1/100; D134-3 MBL International, Woburn, MA), and anti-PDX1 (1/200 in SignalStain antibody diluent; obtained from Christopher V.E., Germany). On the following day, slides were washed 3 x 5 minutes with wash buffer and secondary anti-rat in goat Alexa Fluor 488 nM (1/300; A11006 Invitrogen) or anti-rabbit in goat Alexa Fluor 568 nM (1/300; A11036 Invitrogen) antibody was applied for 1 h at approximately 25°C. An additional blocking step for 30 min at approximately 25°C was performed with blocking solution between the first secondary antibody and the second primary antibody incubation. Finally, the slides were washed, covered with DAPI containing mounting medium (H-1200 Vector Laboratories) and analyzed by fluorescence microscopy (Axiostar Plus FL, Carl Zeiss).

4.3.5 Detection of GFP-LC3 puncta

GFP-LC3 transgenic mice were sacrificed after standard fed conditions or after withholding food for 12-18 h in order to stimulate autophagy. Cryo-sections were air dried, fixed in 100% ethanol for 8 minutes at approximately 25°C, washed with PBS and covered with DAPI containing mounting medium. Sections were processed and kept in the dark until analysis. Puncta formation was detected by analysis of green fluorescence (EX/EM 470/525 nm)

4.3.6 Detection of Cre-Recombinase expression

The expression pattern of Atg5 in *A5* and *ElaCRe;A5* mice, was assessed in Tom-GFP *A5* mice or Tom-GFP *ElaCre;A5* mice older than 18 weeks or 9 weeks respectively. Pancreatic tissue cryo-sections were air-dried and processed as described above (4.3.5). Sections were kept in the dark until analysis. Fluorescence microscopy was used for analysis of Tomato (EX/EM 554/581 nm) and GFP (EX/EM 470/525 nm) expression.

4.3.7 Detection of Reactive Oxygen Species (ROS)

Freshly cut pancreatic tissue cryo-sections were processed as described (4.3.5) and incubated with 20 µM of 2',7'-dichlorofluorescin diacetate

(DCF-DA; D6883 Sigma) in PBS for 30 min at approximately 25°C. Following careful washing with PBS, slides were covered with Fluoromount aqueous mounting medium (F4680 Sigma) and analyzed using fluorescence microscopy (EX/EM 488/530 nm).

4.3.8 Quantification of relative acinar cell area

Paraffin-embedded tissue sections from 18-week old $A5$ and $A5^{F/F}$ mice fed a SD or POD, or treated with NAC-containing drinking water were stained for H&E (4.3.2) and photographed at 100x magnification. The area (μm^2) occupied by acinar cells only and the complete pancreatic area (excluding major islets and blood vessels) was quantified using a proprietary software package (Zeiss Axiovision, Oberkochen, Germany). Measurements from multiple photographs per tissue slide were added and the acinar cell area was expressed relative to the complete area of pancreatic tissue. Results were averaged according to genotype and treatment group and compared to $A5^{F/F}$ mice. By definition, the relative acinar cell area of $A5^{F/F}$ mice was 1 and the relative acinar cell area of other groups was related to this value.

4.3.9 Quantification of proliferation (BrdU) and apoptosis (cleaved caspase 3)

For proliferation analysis, mice were labeled with 50 µg of BrdU (50 µg/µl stock solution in H_2O; B5002, Sigma) per g body weight by i.p. injection and sacrificed 2 h later. The pancreas was fixed and paraffin sections were obtained as described above (4.3.1).

For quantification of acinar cell proliferation and apoptosis in 18-week old $A5$ and $A5^{F/F}$ mice fed a SD or POD, paraffin-embedded tissue sections were stained with anti-BrdU and anti-cleaved caspase 3 as described above (4.3.3). Tissue sections were photographed at 100x or 200x magnification for BrdU and cleaved caspase 3, respectively. The number of positive acinar cells and the area occupied by acinar cells (μm^2) was determined with a proprietary software package (Zeiss Axiovision). The sum of positive acinar cells from multiple photographs per tissue slide was generated and divided by the overall occupied area (positive acinar cells/acinar cell area μm^2). For standardization, results were stated in relation to the average measurement in $A5^{F/F}$ mice.

Quantification of BrdU and cleaved caspase 3 in 4-week old *A5*, *A5;p53*, and *A5;p62* mice was achieved in a manner analogous as described above using 200x magnification. The number of positive acinar cells was determined per high power field and expressed in relation to the average of positive acinar cells per high power field from $A5^{F/F}$ controls.

4.3.10 Transmission Electron microscopy (TEM)

Tissues were fixed in 2.5% electron microscopy grade glutaraldehyde in 0.1 M sodium cacodylate buffer, pH 7.4 (Science Services, Munich, Germany), post-fixed in 2% aqueous osmium tetraoxide *(Dalton, 1955)*, dehydrated in gradual ethanol (30–100%) and propylene oxide, embedded in Epon (Merck), and cured for 24 hours at 60°C. Semithin sections were cut and stained with toluidine blue. Ultrathin sections of 50 nm were collected onto 200 mesh copper grids, stained with uranyl acetate and lead citrate, before examination by TEM (Zeiss Libra 120 Plus, Carl Zeiss NTS GmbH, Oberkochen, Germany). Pictures were acquired using a Slow Scan CCD-camera and iTEM software (Olympus Soft Imaging Solutions, Münster, Germany). TEM sample preparation was done with the help of Gabriele Mettenleiter. TEM image analysis was done with the help of Dr. Michaela Aichler.

4.3.11 Human chronic pancreatitis samples

Pancreatic tissue samples from humans with chronic pancreatitis were collected following pancreatic head resection for CP ($n=8$; male/female=7/1, median age=48yr) as described[35]. The study was reviewed and approved by the ethics committee of the Technische Universität München, and University of Heidelberg, Germany and informed patient consent was obtained for tissue collection. The etiology of CP was alcoholic in all patients. The pancreatic tissue samples were collected under sterile conditions with a median time from cross-clamping to processing of approximately 10-30 min. One portion of the resected pancreatic tissue samples was immediately fixed in 4% PFA followed by paraffin-embedding. p62, Nqo1 and p53 immunohistochemistry was performed as described above (4.3.3).

For transmission electron microscopy, another portion of the pancreatic tissue samples was minced into small pieces, fixed, and processed as described above (4.3.10).

4.4 Proteinbiochemistry

4.4.1 Serum amylase and lipase measurement

Serum was obtained from mice immediately after sacrifice at 4 and 18 weeks of age or after AP induction (0 and 4 h after first cerulein injection) and diluted 1/10 with 0.9% NaCl. Amylase activity (AMYL2 Cobas, Roche) was quantified by a colorimetric assay according to the IFCC method. Lipase activity (LIPC Cobas, Roche) was quantified by DGGR substrate-based assay.

4.4.2 Pancreatic tissue enzyme content and activity

Activity of pancreatic trypsin and cathepsin B were assessed in pancreatic homogenates. For pancreatic tissue homogenization, pancreatic tissue was removed and homogenized in a Potter homogenizer at 2,000 rpm in homogenization buffer (HS buffer: 250 mM sucrose, 10 mM citric acid, 0.5 mM EGTA, 0.1 mM $MgSO_4$, pH 6.0). The homogenate was centrifuged at 200 g for 5 min at 4°C and collected as post-nuclear supernatant. All steps were performed on ice.

Trypsin activity was measured in assay buffer (50 mM Tris-HCl pH 8.0, 150 mM NaCl, 1 mM $CaCl_2$) at 37°C using 32 µM BOC-Gln-Ala-Arg-7-amido-4-methylcoumarin (Bachem, Bubendorf, Switzerland) as fluorogenic substrate and following the kinetic release of 7-amido-4-methylcoumarin in time intervals of 30 seconds over 10 min at the excitation/emission wave length of 360/438 nm in a Safire microplate reader (Tecan, Grödig, Austria). Activity was calculated by measurement of specific enzyme activity of a diluted purified bovine trypsin standard (100 ng/ml final concentration) (Sigma) under identical assay conditions.

Cathepsin B activity was determined as Ca074-sensitive activity using the fluorogenic substrate Z-Phe-Arg-7-amino-4-methylcoumarin (10 µM) (Bachem). Assays were performed in assay buffer (50 mM sodium phosphate buffer, pH 5.5, 1 mM EDTA, 1 mM dithiothreitol). The release of 7-amino-4-methylcoumarin was kinetically monitored by spectrofluorometry. Tissue contents of cathepsin B were calculated using a standard curve of purified human cathepsin B (Calbiochem/Merck). Enzyme contents and activities were measured in the lab of Prof. Walter Halangk with the help of Dr. Thomas Wartmann and Robert Fischer, Otto-von-Guericke Universität, Magdeburg, Germany.

4.4.3 Subcellular fractionation by isopycnic Percoll density centrifugation and measurement of GLDH activity

To analyze mitochondrial integrity and distribution in subcellular fractions pancreatic homogenate (produced as described under 4.4.2) was applied onto an isotonic 50% (v/v) Percoll/HS buffer solution (described under 4.4.2) at pH 7.27. The pancreatic homogenate was subsequently separated by isopycnic centrifugation at 50,000 g for 45 min at 4°C. After separation of mitochondria, the percoll gradient was fractionated in 46 fractions using a peristaltic pump beginning from the bottom and fractions were stored at -80°C until further use.

Activity of GLDH as a marker of mitochondrial distribution in subcellular fractions was determined spectrophotometrically at 340 nm according to $NADH_2$ oxidation with 2-oxoglutarate and NH_4^+ as a substrate by the method of E. Schmidt[36].

Data on GLDH were obtained in the lab of Prof. Walter Halangk with the help of Dr. Thomas Wartmann and Robert Fischer, Otto-von-Guericke Universität Magdeburg, Germany.

4.4.4 Mitochondrial Respiratory Complex II and IV Activity Assays in isolated pancreatic mitochondria

For isolation of pancreatic mitochondria, pancreatic tissue from 4-week old, male *A5* and *A5$^{F/F}$* mice was quickly minced with a sharp blade in ice-cold isolation buffer (300 mM sucrose, 5 mM TES, 0.2 mM EGTA, pH 7.2) supplemented with 0.5% BSA and 4x protease inhibitor cocktail (complete protease inhibitor cocktail tablets, Roche), shortly homogenized (2x 1,000 U/min), and centrifuged twice at 800 g for 10 min at 4°C. Pellet containing cell debris, nuclei, and zymogen granules were discarded and mitochondria were obtained from the supernatant centrifuged at 10,000 g for 10 min at 4°C. After washing the mitochondria two times (10,000 g, 10 min, 4°C), wherein BSA and protease inhibitors, which could adversely affect respiratory complex function, were left out in the last washing step, mitochondria were carefully resuspended in isolation buffer and the protein concentration was estimated by Bradford. Isolation of pancreatic mitochondria was performed in the lab of Dr. Hans Zischka with the help of Josef Lichtmanegger, Helmholtz Zentrum, Munich, Germany.

For Complex IV activity, mitochondria were diluted to 0.04 mg/ml with Tris/KCl buffer (120 mM KCl, 50 mM Tris-HCl, pH 7.4) and kept on ice. Measurements were performed in triplicates with 2 µg mitochondria per well. The reaction buffer per well contained Tris/KCl buffer (120 mM KCl, 50 mM Tris-HCl, pH 7.4) and 2.5 mM β-dodecyl-D-maltoside. Oxidation of ferrocytochrome C (22 µM per well, produced by reduction of ferricytochrome C (C2037, Sigma; 95%, 8,9% H_2O)) was assessed spectrophotometrically in 6 second intervals at a wavelength of 550 nm absorption and 37°C for a total of 1 min. Activity (nmol/min/mg) was determined by calculating the slope of the linear part of the resulting curve (absorption/min), multiplied by 5552.16 (factor determined by sample volume and plate well diameter). Activities of negative controls (treated with 50-250 mM potassium cyanide per well) were subtracted from each sample.

For Complex II activity, mitochondria were diluted to 1 mg/ml with 25 mM dipotassium hydrogen phosphate buffer (pH 7.4) and kept on ice. Measurements were performed in triplicates with 20 µg mitochondria per well. The reaction buffer per well contained 25 mM dipotassium hydrogen phosphate buffer (pH 7.4), 2.5 mM β-dodecyl-D-maltoside, 20 mM succinate, 2 mM potassium cyanide, 50 µM dichlorphenolindophenole, 2 µg/µl rotenone and 2 µg/µl antimycine A.

Oxidation of decylubiquinone (56 µM per well, BML-CM115-0050, Enzo, Siegburg, Germany) was assessed spectrophotometrically in 10 second intervals at a wavelength of 600 nm and 37°C for a total of 10 min. Activity (nmol/min/mg) was determined by calculating the slope of the linear part of the resulting curve (absorption/min), multiplied by 844.45 (factor determined by sample volume and plate well diameter). Negative controls included thenoyltrifluoracetone (0.11 mg/ml per well).
Measurement of C II and C IV activities was performed by Yashar Kabiri in the lab of Dr. Hans Zischka, Helmholtz Zentrum Munich, Germany.

4.4.5 Protein extraction and quantification

Protein extraction was performed on ice. Snap frozen tissue samples were homogenized, sonicated (2 x 10 sec), and lysed in ice-cold protein lysis buffer (IP-buffer: 50 mM HEPES, pH 7.9, 150 mM NaCl, 1 mM EDTA, pH 8.0, 0.5% (v/v) NP-40, 10% (v/v) Glycerol) freshly supplemented with a cocktail of protease (2% (v/v))/phosphatase (1% (v/v)) inhibitors (SERVA, Heidelberg, Germany). Homogenates were incubated for 30 min at 4°C and subsequently centrifuged (13,000 rpm, 30 min, 4°C). Supernatants were collected and centrifuged again (13,000 rpm, 5 min, 4°C) to ensure complete removal of cell debris. Protein concentration was estimated from a 1/10 dilution of the supernatant in IP-buffer with the Bio Rad Protein Assay Kit (Bio Rad, München, Germany) by mixing 200 µl Bio Rad Protein Assay Kit (diluted 1/5 in H_2O) with 2 µl protein dilution in a 96-well plate. BSA (1 mg/ml; Sigma) was used as a standard and IP-buffer was used as blank. Following a 10 min incubation at approximately 25°C, extinction at 595 nm was measured and protein concentration was determined by the standard curve. Samples were subsequently adjusted to 4 µg/µl with 5 x Laemmli buffer (300 mM Tris-HCl, pH 6.8, 10% (w/v) SDS, 50% (v/v) Glycerol,

0.05% (w/v) Bromphenole blue, 5% (v/v) β-mercaptoethanol), heated (5 min, 95°C), cooled down, centrifuged shortly and stored at -80°C until further use.

4.4.6 SDS-PAGE

SDS-polyacrylamide gel electrophoresis for protein separation and subsequent western blot analysis was performed in a Mini-Protean® 3 Cell System (Bio Rad). 50-80 µg protein per sample (depending on the protein of interest) in Laemmli-buffer (described above (4.4.5)) were denatured by heating at 95°C for 5 min. After cooling down at approximately 25°C and a short centrifugation, proteins were loaded onto the gel. A protein standard (Bio Rad) was used to determine kDa-size of the proteins. The gel consisted of an upper Collection gel (10% polyacrylamide concentration) and a lower Separating gel (7.5-15% polyacrylamide concentration depending on protein size). Gel run was performed in Running buffer at 70 V for 20 min followed by 90-120 V (depending on polyacrylamide concentration) until protein separation (depending on the size of the protein). Table 8 describes the detailed components of the buffers used for SDS-PAGE and Table 9 and 10 describe how the gels were poured.

Table 8: Detailed components of buffers used for SDS-PAGE.

Name	Components	pH
Collection gel buffer	0.5 mM Tris	6.8
Separating gel buffer	1.5 mM Tris	8.8
Running buffer	25 mM Tris-HCL, 192 mM Glycine, 0.1% (w/v) SDS	Not measured

Table 9: Components of SDS-Collection gels.

dH_2O	3.0 ml
Collection gel buffer	1.3 ml
30%/0.8% Acrylamide/Bis solution (Roth, Karlsruhe, Germany)	750 µl
10% SDS	50 µl
10% APS (Sigma)	25 µl
TEMED (Fluka, Buchs, Schweiz)	10 µl

Table 10: Components of SDS-Separating gels according to varying polyacrylamide concentration.

Separating gel	7.5%	10%	12%	15%
dH_2O	4.9 ml	4.1 ml	3.4 ml	2.5 ml
Separating gel buffer	2.6 ml	2.6 ml	2.6 ml	2.6 ml
30%/0.8% Acrylamide/Bis solution	2.5 ml	3.3 ml	4.0 ml	5.0 ml
10% SDS	100 µl	100 µl	100 µl	100 µl
10% APS	50 µl	50 µl	50 µl	50 µl
TEMED	15 µl	15 µl	15 µl	15 µl

4.4.7 Western blot

After SDS-PAGE (4.4.6), proteins were transferred onto a PVDF membrane (0.45 or 0.2 µm pore size, Merck Millipore) by western blot in the Mini Trans-Blot Cell™ System (Bio Rad). PVDF membranes were hydrophilized prior to usage in 100% methanol for 1 min, followed by washing in water and Transfer buffer (Table 11). Western blot was performed in Transfer buffer (pre-cooled to 4°C) on ice at 390 mA for 1-2 h (depending on protein size). After transfer, membranes were washed shortly in TBS-T or PBS-T (Table 7) and incubated for 1 h at approximately 25°C on a shaker in blocking solution (Table 11) to block unspecific binding of the antibodies. Primary antibody incubation was performed in antibody solution (Table 11) for 12-18 h at 4°C on a shaker. The primary antibodies used included: anti-Atg5 (1/1000; NB110-53818, Novus Biologicals, Heford, Germany), anti-p62 (1/1000; GP62-C, Progen), anti-LC3 (1/1000; PD014, MBL International), anti-phosho-CREB (1/1000; 9191, Cell Signaling Technology), anti-CREB (1/1000; 9197, Cell Signaling Technology), anti-CPA (1/1000; 1810-0006, AbD Serotec), anti-ubiquitin (1/1000; BML-PW8810, Enzo), anti-PMP70 (1/1000; SP5237P, Acris), anti-Lamp2 (1/1000; 51-2200, ZYMED Laboratories, Carlsbad, CA), anti-HSP90 (1/1000; sc-7947, Santa Cruz), anti-Erk1 (1/1000; sc-93, Santa Cruz), anti-Erk2 (1/1000; sc-154, Santa Cruz), and anti-β-Actin (1/2000; A5441, Sigma). Following incubation, membranes were washed 3 x 5 min with TBS-T or PBS-T and the secondary antibody was added in antibody solution (Table 11) (horseradish peroxidase-conjugated anti-mouse (1/5000; NA931V GE Healthcare), anti-rabbit (1/10000; NA934V GE Healthcare), or anti-guinea pig (1/5000; A7289, Sigma)) for 1 h at approximately 25°C on a shaker. Prior to development, membranes were washed again 2 x 10 min with TBS-T or PBS-T and 1 x 5 min with TBS or PBS. Development was performed with the Amersham ECL™ western blot detection reagent (GE Healthcare, Buckinghamshire, UK) and the Amersham Hyperfilm™ ECL (GE Healthcare). Exposure of films to membranes varied (2 sec-2 h) depending on the signal obtained from the protein of interest.

Table 11: Components of solutions used for western blot.

Name	Components
Transfer buffer	25 mM Tris-HCl, 192 mM Glycine, 20% (v/v) Methanol
Blocking solution	5% BSA or 5-10% milk in TBS-T or PBS-T (depending on antibody)
Antibody solution	2% BSA or 2% milk in TBS-T or PBS-T (depending on antibody)

4.5 Metabolomics and Lipidomics

4.5.1 Non-targeted metabolomics profiling

Frozen mouse pancreatic tissue weighing approximately 29 to 55 mg were weighed and placed into pre-cooled (dry ice) 2 ml homogenization tubes containing ceramic beads with a diameter of 1.4 mm. Pre-cooled water was added based on tissue weight at 5 µl/mg tissue. The samples were then homogenized using a Precellys 24 homogenizer (Peqlab) equipped with an integrated cooling unit three times for 20 s at 5500 rpm, with 30 s intervals (to ensure freezing temperature in the sample vials) between the homogenization cycles. After homogenization, 100 µl of the homogenate were loaded onto 96-well 2 ml deep plates. In addition to the study samples, a pooled human reference plasma sample and a pooled sample of all homogenates from this study were extracted independently one and three per 96-well plate, respectively. These samples served as control replicates throughout the study to assess process variability. Besides the reference plasma samples, 100 µl of water were extracted independently three per 96-well plate to serve as blanks. The samples in the 96-well plate were extracted with 475 µl methanol, containing four recovery standards to monitor the extraction efficiency. After centrifugation, the supernatant was split into 4 aliquots. The first 2 aliquots were used for LC/MS analysis in both positive and negative electrospray ionization mode. Two further aliquots on the second plate were kept as a reserve. The samples were dried on a TurboVap 96 (Zymark, Sotax, Lörrach, Germany). Prior to LC/MS in positive ion mode, the samples were reconstituted with 100 µl of 0.1% formic acid. Those samples analyzed in negative ion mode were reconstituted with 100 µl of 6.5 mM ammonium bicarbonate, pH 8.0. Reconstitution solvents for both ionization modes contained internal standards that allowed monitoring of instrument performance and also served as retention markers. LC/MS analysis was performed on a linear ion trap LTQ XL mass spectrometer (Thermo Fisher Scientific) coupled with a Waters Acquity UPLC system (Waters GmbH, Eschborn, Germany). Two separate columns (2.1 x 100 mm Waters BEH C18, 1.7 µm particle-size) were used for acidic (solvent A: 0.1% formic acid in water, solvent B: 0.1% formic acid in methanol) and for basic (solvent A: 6.5 mM ammonium bicarbonate, pH 8.0, solvent B: 6.5 mM ammonium bicarbonate in 95% methanol) mobile phase conditions, optimized for positive and negative electrospray ionization, respectively. After injection of the sample extracts, the columns were developed with a gradient of 99.5% A to 98% B over an 11 min run time at a flow rate of 350 µl/min. The eluent flow was directly routed through the ESI source of the LTQ XL mass spectrometer. The full MS scan was performed from 80 to 1000 m/z and alternated between MS and MS/MS scans using a dynamic exclusion technique, which enables a wide range of metabolite coverage.

Metabolites detected were annotated by curation of the LC-MS/MS data against Metabolon's chemical database library (Metabolon, Inc., Durnham, NC, USA) based on retention index, precursor mass, and MS/MS spectra. In this study, 264 known metabolites and 79 compounds with an unknown chemical structure, indicated by the letter X followed by a number as the compound identifier, were identified. The area under the curve was normalized to the median of each identified metabolite for each of the days the assay was performed to correct for inter-day variation of the measurements. The metabolites were assigned to cellular pathways based on PubChem, KEGG, and the Human Metabolome Database (HMDB). Metabolic pathways were described as significantly up- or downregulated, when metabolites assigned to those specific pathways were increased or decreased, respectively. Data was obtained at the Institute of Experimental Genetics and at the Institute of Bioinformatics and Systems Biology, Helmholtz Zentrum Munich, Germany, in the in the lab of Prof. Jerzy Adamski with the help of Dr. Anna Artati and in the lab of Dr. Werner Roemisch-Margl respectively.

4.5.2 Characterization of mitochondrial cardiolipin composition

CL-extraction: CL was extracted from the samples by a modified Folch extraction procedure[37]. 50 ng of tetra-myristoyl-CL ((C14:0)4-CL; Avanti Polar Lipids Inc., Alabaster, AL) was added as an internal standard to 10 µl mitochondrial suspension. Chloroform/methanol (2/1, v/v) containing 0.05% BHT as antioxidant was added. The lipid and aqueous phases were separated by adding 0.01 M HCl, followed by intensive shaking, and centrifugation. After centrifugation, the lower lipid phase was collected and dried under nitrogen atmosphere and acidified. Ice-cold methanol (2 ml), chloroform (1 ml), and 0.1 M HCl (1 ml) were added and the solution was intensively mixed. After 5 min of incubation on ice the samples were separated by the addition of chloroform (1 ml) and 0.1 M HCl (1 ml). The chloroform/methanol phase was recovered as CL-containing sample. The samples were dried under nitrogen and dissolved in 0.8 ml chloroform/methanol/water (50/45/5, v/v/v). After mixing and filtering of the mixture over 0.2 µm PTFE membranes the samples were ready for analysis.

HPLC–MS/MS analysis: Molecular CL species were analyzed as previously described[38] with minor modifications. For the analysis of CL a TSQ Quantum Discovery Max (Thermo Fisher Scientific) was used in the negative ion electrospray ionization (ESI) mode. The HPLC system consisted of a Surveyor MS quaternary narrow bore pump with integrated vacuum degasser and a Surveyor auto sampler. Auto sampler tray temperature was held at 8°C. In partial loop mode a sample of 10 µl of lipid extract dissolved in chloroform/methanol/water (50/45/5, v/v/v) was injected and CL was separated by using a LiChroCart column (125 mm × 2 mm), LiChrospher Si60 (5 µm particle diameter; Merck) and a linear gradient of solution A (chloroform with 25% aqueous ammonia (0.1 ml/l)) and solution B (methanol/water 9:1, v/v with 25% aqueous ammonia (0.1 ml/l)). The gradient was as follows: 0–0.2 min 92% solution A, 8% solution B; 0.2–4.5 min 92–30% solution A, 8–70% solution B; 4.5–6 min 30% solution A, 70% solution B; 6–6.5 min 30–92% solution A, 70–8% solution B; and 6.5–11 min 92% solution A, 8% solution B. The flow rate was 200 µl/min. Total time of analysis was 11 min. The eluate collected between 0.3 and 6 min was analyzed by mass spectrometry. Nitrogen was used as the nebulizing gas and argon as collision gas at a pressure of 1.5 mTorr. The spray voltage was 3.5 kV, the ion source capillary temperature was set at 375°C and the cone-voltage was 30 V. Daughter fragments from the doubly charged parent derived from $(C18:2)_4$-CL with m/z 723.6 $((M-2H)^{2-}/2)$ were obtained using a collision energy of 36 eV. This molecular CL species and the internal standard (m/z 619.6) were analyzed by mass transfer reaction monitoring their doubly charged ions and their respective fatty acids linoleic acid m/z 279.2 and myristic acid m/z 227.2 using the selected reaction monitoring (SRM) mode. The same approach was used for parent and daughter fragments of other molecular species of CL. The quantity of these molecular species was related to the content of (C18:2)$_4$-CL. Oxidized CL ((C18:2)$_3$-monohydroxylinoleic acid-CL) was measured in the SRM mode as a transition from m/z 731.6 to m/z 279.2 (linoleic acid) as previously described[39]. Data were obtained and analyzed by Prof. Lorenz Schild, Otto-von-Guericke Universität, Magdeburg, Germany.

4.6 Statistics

Data are displayed as averages ± standard deviations (SD). Parameters for the groups were compared by Mann-Whitney test or two-sided Student's t-tests as appropriate and statistical significance was set at *P<0.05, **P<0.01, ***P<0.001. The statistical software Prism 5 (GraphPad Software, Inc.) was used for analysis.

5 RESULTS

5.1 Autophagy in the pancreas

5.1.1 Baseline and starvation induced autophagy

Starvation is a known inducer of autophagy *in vivo*[34]. In order to verify that autophagy is inducible in the pancreas, mice were starved for 18h and compared to fed mice (Figure 4). Indeed, starvation increased LC3 II protein-levels, as measured by western blot (Figure 4A) and GFP-LC3-positive puncta (Figure 4B) in pancreatic tissue of wildtype and *GFP-LC3* mice respectively.

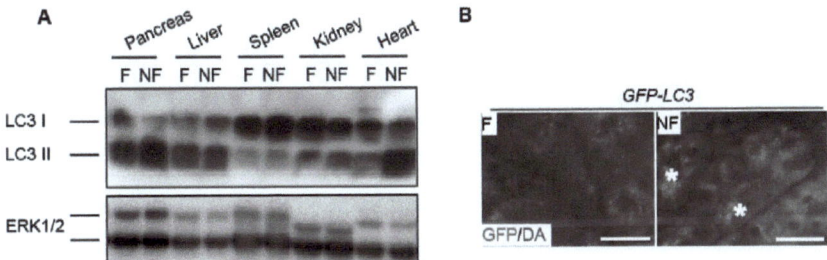

Figure 4: Autophagy is detectable and inducible in the pancreas. (A) Detection of LC3 I/II by western blot analysis of pancreatic, liver, spleen, kidney and heart lysates from fed (F) and non-fed (NF) mice; ERK1 and 2 were used as loading controls. (B) Autophagy stimulation in the pancreas of *GFP-LC3* transgenic mice in response to being fed (F, left) and compared to having food withheld (NF, right); GFP-positive dots represent autophagosomes (white asterisk); nuclei are stained with DAPI (DA); scale bars equal 10 µm.

Thus, autophagy was detectable and inducible in the pancreas. Interestingly, pancreatic tissue exhibited one of the highest degrees of LC3-lipidation compared to other organs (Figure 4A), further highlighting the relevance of autophagy in pancreatic homeostasis.

5.1.2 Acute pancreatitis and autophagy

To further characterize pancreatic autophagy, autophagy under experimental AP conditions was analyzed. AP was induced in *GFP-LC3* transgenic mice, following a 4h, 8h and 3 day protocol respectively. GFP-LC3 puncta were detectable at all three time-points (Figure 5). Increased puncta formation was observed after 8h and 3 days, indicative of more autophagosome formation.

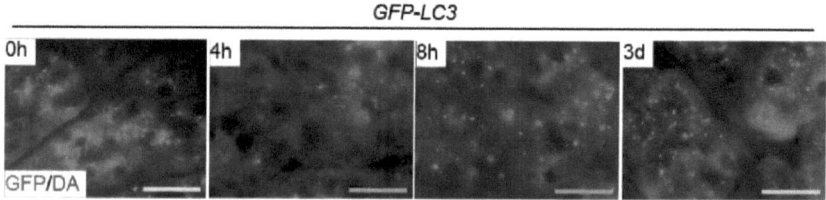

Figure 5: Acute pancreatitis stimulates autophagosome formation. Detection of GFP-LC3 positive puncta in the pancreas of *GFP-LC3* transgenic mice at baseline (0h) and after acute pancreatitis induction (4h, 8h, 3 days); nuclei are stained with DAPI (DA); scale bars equal 10 μm.

Thus, autophagy was induced in the pancreas upon AP-mediated acinar cell stress.

5.2 Pancreas-specific inactivation of autophagy

5.2.1 *A5* mice exhibit features of CP

Past studies have associated autophagy with pancreatic homeostasis and disease. Nevertheless, results remain conflicting and precise evidence is lacking. Indeed, while conditional inactivation of *Atg5* in acinar cells resulted in no overt phenotype[40], impaired autophagy has been described in pancreatitis[24]. In order to elucidate the role of pancreatic autophagy, pancreas-specific autophagy deficient mice were generated and analyzed at various time-points after birth. Embryonic loss of Atg5 in *Ptf1aCre^ex1;Atg5^F/F* (termed A5) mice blocked pancreatic autophagy, as shown by accumulation of LC3 I and p62 in the pancreas but not in the liver of A5 mice (Figure 6).

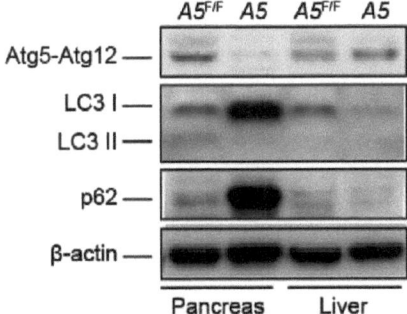

Figure 6: Block of pancreatic autophagy in A5 mice. Detection of Atg5-Atg12, LC3 I/II and p62 in the pancreas and liver of A5 and A5^F/F control mice by western blot; β-actin was used as loading control.

Blocked autophagic degradation resulted in edematous and enlarged pancreata at 4 weeks of age (Figure 7A), with acinar cells exhibiting extensive cytoplasmic vacuolization (Figure 7B). As A5 mice grew older, pancreata became atrophic (Figure 7A, C). Importantly, numerous duct-like structures appeared throughout the pancreas and remaining acinar cells acquired a hypertrophic phenotype (Figure 7B). Simultaneously, A5 mice exhibited a significant decrease in body weight, indicative of cachexia (Figure 7D).

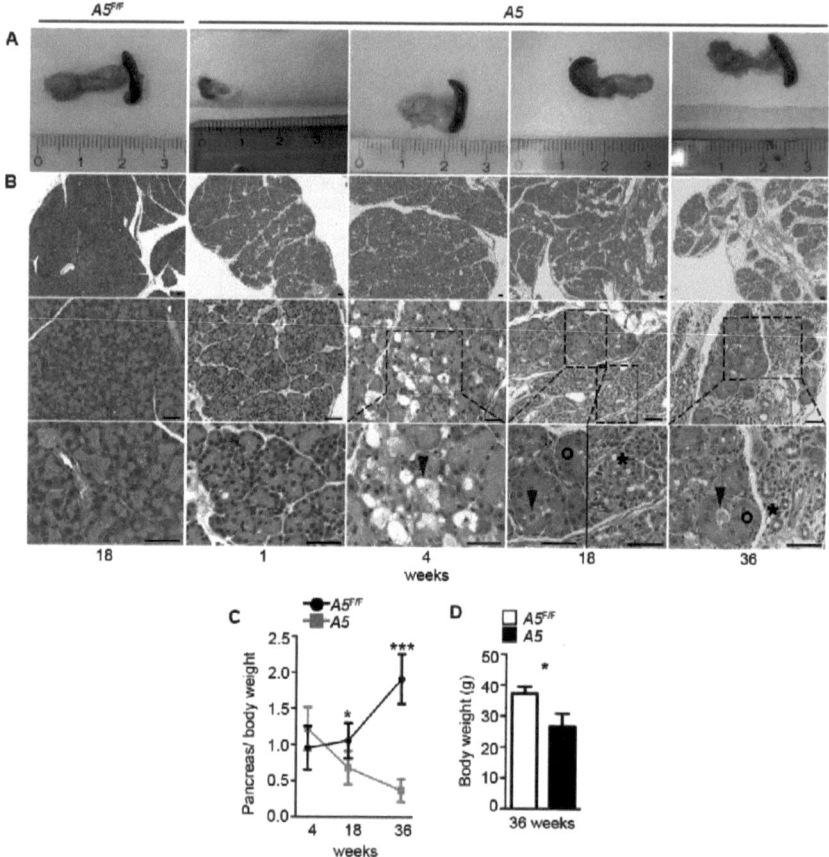

Figure 7: Pancreas-specific autophagy deficiency results in exocrine pancreatic degeneration. (**A**) Macroscopic and (**B**) microscopic (H&E) appearance of pancreata from 1/4/18/36-week old Atg5 deficient mice (A5) compared to that of 18-week old floxed control mice ($A5^{F/F}$); arrowhead, asterisk, and circle indicate vacuolization, duct-like structures, and hypertrophic acinar cells, respectively; scale bars equal 50 μm. (**C**) Pancreas/body weight over time in $A5^{F/F}$ (black line, black circle) and A5 (red line, red square) mice; means±SD (n≥3), *P<0.05, ***P<0.001. (**D**) Body weight (g) of 36-week old male $A5^{F/F}$ (open bar) and A5 (black bar) mice; means±SD (n≥3), *P<0.05.

Heterozygous $A5^{F/-}$ mice, on the other hand, appeared normal at all time-points analyzed (Figure 8). Moreover, defects due to autophagy deficiency seemed to develop postnatally, since no defects were visible in A5 mice at 1 week of age (Figure 7A).

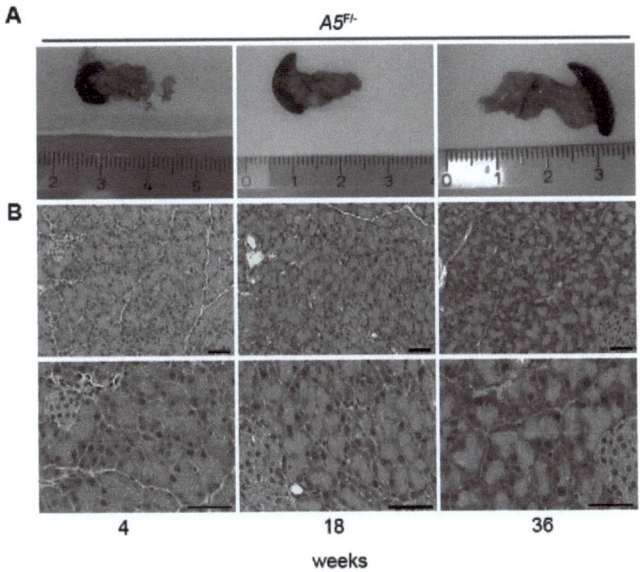

Figure 8: Heterozygous $A5^{F/-}$ mice display normal pancreatic morphology. (A) Macroscopic and (B) microscopic (H&E) appearance of pancreata from 4/18/36-week old Atg5 heterozygous mice ($A5^{F/-}$); scale bars equal 50 μm.

Further characterization of A5 mice revealed multiple hallmark features of CP. Serum lipase activity (Figure 9A) and pancreatic tissue trypsin (Figure 9B) and cathepsin B (Figure 9C) activities were significantly increased in 4-week old A5 mice. In addition, carboxypeptidase A (CPA), an enzyme involved in polypeptide breakdown and a major component of pancreatic juice[41], was found cleaved in protein lysates of A5 pancreas (Figure 9D). CPA is cleaved and activated by pancreatic digestive enzymes[41], thus cleavage of CPA is indicative of increased pancreatic enzyme activity. Moreover, A5 mice exhibited increased fibrosis, inflammation, proliferation, apoptosis, and necrosis (Figure 9E).

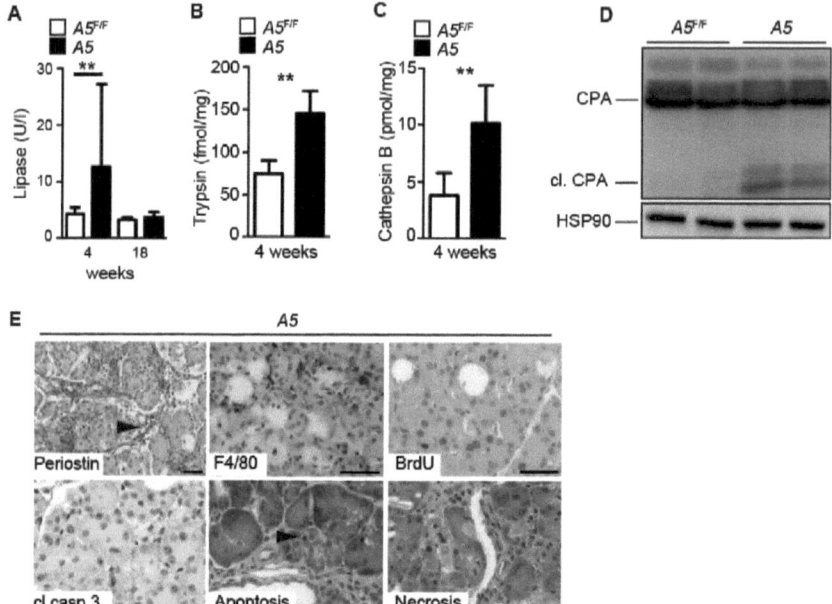

Figure 9: A5 mice display features of CP. (**A**) Serum lipase activities (U/l) in A5 (black bar) compared to $A5^{F/F}$ (open bar) at 4 (n=10 per group) and 18 (n=8 A5, n=3 $A5^{F/F}$) weeks of age; means±SD, **P<0.01. (**B**) Amounts of activated trypsin (fmol/mg) and (**C**) cathepsin B (pmol/mg) in the pancreas of 4-week old A5 (black bar) mice as compared to controls (open bar); units are per mg pancreatic protein, means±SD, (n≥6), **P<0.01. (**D**) Western blot analysis of carboxypeptidase A/cleaved carboxypeptidase A (CPA/cl. CPA) in pancreatic lysates of 4-week old $A5^{F/F}$ and A5 mice; HSP90 was used as loading control. (**E**) Histological and immunohistochemical analyses for fibrosis (periostin, black arrowhead), inflammation (F4/80), proliferation (BrdU), apoptosis (cleaved caspase 3 (cl. casp 3) and H&E with black arrowhead), and necrosis (H&E) in A5 pancreas; scale bars equal 50 μm.

Taken together, pancreas-specific autophagy deficiency closely mirrored all stages of CP, including detrimental organ damage, inflammation, fibrosis, and degeneration.

5.2.2 Adult acinar cells are resistant to autophagy deficiency

The only study so far utilizing pancreas-specific autophagy-deficient mice did not report any morphological alterations; the study even showed rescue of cerulein-induced AP in *Atg5*-deficient mice[40]. However, the authors examined mice with knockout of *Atg5* in mature and not embryonic acinar cells. In order to assess the role of autophagy in mature acinar cells, $A5^{F/F}$ mice were crossed with mice expressing Cre recombinase under the tamoxifen-inducible *Elastase* promoter (termed *ElaCre;A5*). Elastase is expressed only in mature acinar cells and tamoxifen triggers Cre-activation with subsequent *Atg5* excision. Induction of Cre recombinase expression in *ElaCre;A5* mice (Figure 10A) resulted in approximately 70% of acinar cells carrying homozygous deletion of *Atg5*, as revealed by lineage tracing (Figure 10B). Western blotting of Atg5-Atg12, p62 and LC3I/II confirmed loss of Atg5 and blocked autophagic flux in *ElaCre;A5* pancreata. Accumulation of p62, however, was less compared to *A5* pancreata (Figure 10C). Macroscopic differences were not visible (Figure 10D); however careful microscopic examination revealed areas of acinar cell stress at 9 weeks of age (Figure 10E). At 18 weeks of age morphological changes compared to wildtype were minimal, although some inflammatory areas were detectable (Figure 10E).

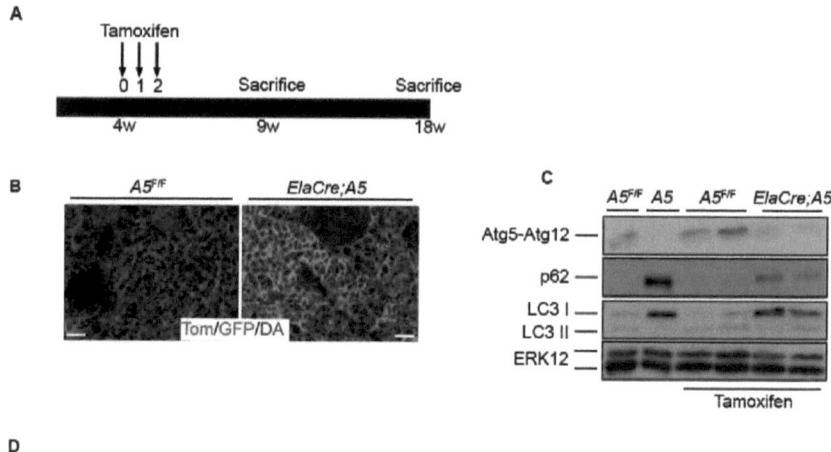

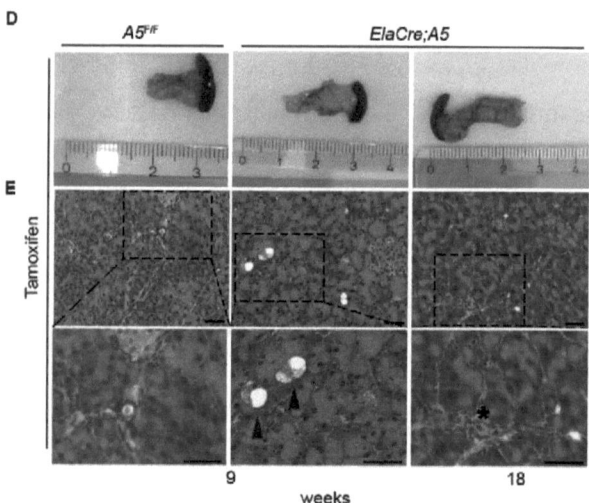

Figure 10: Adult acinar cells are resistant to autophagy deficiency. (**A**) Scheme illustrating induction of Cre-recombinase expression in 4-week old *Elastase-Cre* expressing A5 mice (*ElaCre;A5*) by tamoxifen injection at day 0, 1 and 2; mice were sacrificed at 9 and 18 weeks of age. (**B**) Representative Tomato/GFP immunofluorescence of Tomato-GFP expressing $A5^{F/F}$ (left) and *ElaCre;A5* (right) mice; nuclei are stained with DAPI (DA); scale bars equal 50 μm. (**C**) Atg5-Atg12, p62 and LC3I/II expression in tamoxifen treated *ElaCre;A5* and $A5^{F/F}$ mice compared to untreated $A5^{F/F}$ and A5 mice; ERK1 and 2 were used as loading controls. (**D**) Macroscopic and (**E**) microscopic (H&E) appearance of tamoxifen-treated $A5^{F/F}$ and *ElaCre;A5* mice at 9 and 18 weeks of age; arrowheads and asterisk indicate vacuolization and inflammation respectively; scale bars equal 50 μm.

Furthermore, AP was induced in *ElaCre;A5* and *A5$^{F/F}$* mice to analyze acinar cell stress-resistance. Interestingly, no morphological difference was observed between *ElaCre;A5* and control mice (Figure 11).

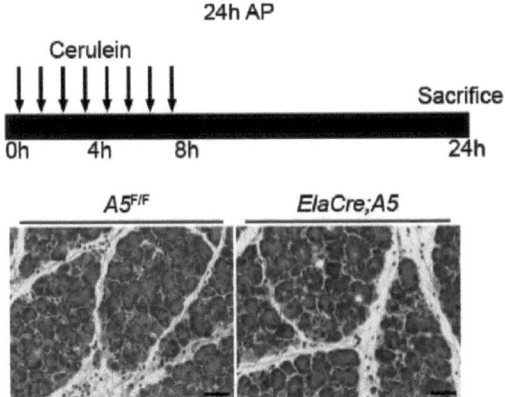

Figure 11. Loss of autophagy in adult acinar cells does not influence pancreatic morphology after AP-induction. Induction of 24 h acute pancreatitis (AP) in *ElaCre;A5* and *A5$^{F/F}$* mice; (top) experimental scheme illustrating hourly, intraperitoneal cerulein injection starting from 0 h and ending at 8 h, including a total of 8 injections; mice were sacrificed 24 h after the first injection; (bottom) microscopic (H&E) examination of *ElaCre;A5* and *A5$^{F/F}$* mice; scale bars equal 50 µm.

Concluding, *Atg5*-deletion in mature versus embryonic acinar cells resulted in a less severe pancreatic phenotype.

5.2.3 Persistent acinar-to-ductal metaplasia in *A5* mice

Exocrine pancreatic injury is compensated by various regeneration mechanisms, recapitulating in part embryonic development[42-45]. Depending on the severity of injury[42] transdifferentiation, dedifferentiation, or simple expansion of acinar cells can occur. Additionally, ductal cells and pancreas-specific adult stem cells, also known as terminal duct cells/centroacinar cells, are capable of renewing exocrine pancreatic tissue. In order to characterize in more detail the tubular structures found in *A5* mice at 18 and 36 weeks of age, lineage tracing with Tomato-GFP expressing *A5* mice was performed. Acinar cells as wells as tubular structures were GFP and therefore Ptf1a positive, implying that both cell types retained loss of functional Atg5 (Figure 12A). On the other hand, stromal cells surrounding tubular structures were Tomato positive and Ptf1a negative (Figure 12A). In addition, tubular structures were found to be positive for ductal markers CK19, HNF1β and SOX9, while remaining negative for the terminal duct/centroacinar cell marker Hes1 and the embryonic marker PDX1 (Figure 12B). Interestingly, regenerative areas also exhibited occasional amylase/CK19 double-positivity (Figure 12B). Moreover, relative expression of digestive enzymes *amylase* and *elastase* as well as of the acinar cell-specific transcription factor *Bhlha15* (known as *Mist1*) significantly decreased (Figure 12C). Relative expression of the ductal marker *Hnf1b*, on the other hand, increased (Figure 12C).

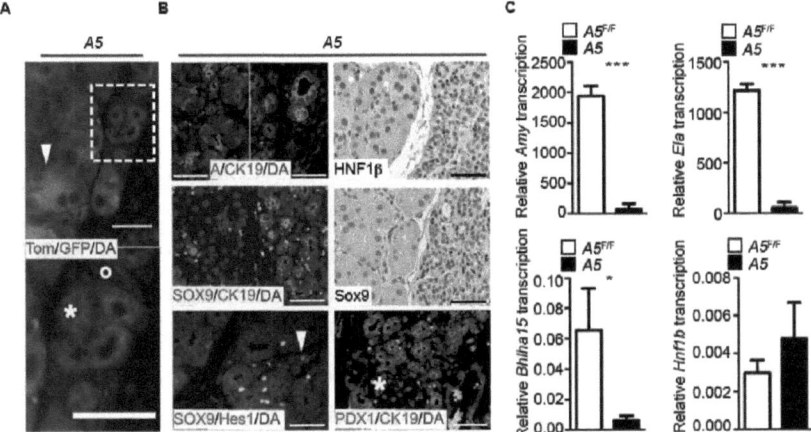

Figure 12: A5 mice exhibit persistent acinar-to-ductal metaplasia. (A) Lineage tracing of duct-like structures in 18-week old Tomato (Tom)-GFP expressing A5 mice; white arrowhead, asterisk and circle indicate GFP-positive acinar cell, GFP-positive duct-like cells and Tom-positive stromal cells; duct-like structures are marked by a box in the top frame and are magnified in the bottom frame; nuclei are stained with DAPI (DA); scale bars equal 50 μm. (B) Immunofluorescence (Amylase (A)/CK19, SOX9/CK19, SOX9/Hes1, PDX1/CK19) and immunohistochemical (HNF1β, SOX9) staining of pancreata from 18-week old A5 mice; white arrowhead and asterisk indicate SOX9/Hes1 positive cell and PDX1-positive/CK19-negative islet respectively; nuclei are stained with DAPI (DA); scale bars equal 50 μm. (C) Relative transcription of acinar cell markers *amylase* (*Amy*), *elastase* (*Ela*), and *Mist1* (*Bhlha15*) and ductal marker *Hnf1b* in whole pancreata of 18-week old A5 mice (black bars) compared to $A5^{F/F}$ controls (open bars); data are normalized to *Cyclophilin*; means±SD, (n=3), *P<0.05, ***P<0.001.

In summary, chronic damage of the exocrine pancreas upon autophagy deficiency initiated a regenerative program leading to accumulation of tubular structures with ductal but not acinar, embryonic or stem cell markers. Importantly, occasional amylase/CK19 co-expression supported a process of acinar-to-ductal metaplasia.

5.2.4 Whole genome transcriptomics and non-targeted metabolomics

Previous results suggest a role of Atg5-dependent autophagy in development of CP. In the following section, whole-genome transcriptomics and non-targeted metabolomics were performed to uncover mechanisms underlying phenotypic alterations in A5 mice.

Gene enrichment analysis using KEGG database revealed multiple upregulated signaling pathways in 4 and 18-week old male A5 mice (Figure 13A). Normalized enrichment score versus significance plots indicated upregulation of 153 and 157 pathways in 4 and 18-week old A5 mice respectively, compared to 20 and 16 in the corresponding wildtype controls (Figure 13A). Among the upregulated gene sets 90 and 87 were significantly enriched in 4 and 18-week old A5 mice respectively compared to 1 in both 4 and 18-week old control mice (Figure 13A).

Highly significant gene sets were further divided into categories based on KEGG pathway description (Figure 13B and Figure 14). Immune signaling, ROS and cell homeostasis (e.g., DNA replication, apoptosis etc.) associated pathways were enriched in both 4- and 18-week old A5 mice (Figure 13B). Differentially affected were pathways involved in cell stress (e.g., mismatch repair, RNA degradation etc.), extracellular matrix, and metabolism (i.e., amino sugar and nucleotide sugar metabolism) (Figure 13B). Direct comparison of highly significant gene sets between the age groups revealed 13, 32 and 3 pathways that were specifically enriched only in 4-week old, both in 4 and 18-week old or only in 18-week old A5 mice respectively (Figure 13C and Figure 14). Among the commonly induced gene sets were pathways like chemokine and T cell receptor signaling, apoptosis, lysosome, and endocytosis (Figure 13C). Gene sets enriched in only 4-or 18 -week old A5 mice included cell cycle, p53 signaling, glutathione metabolism or antigen processing and presentation respectively (Figure 13C). Part of the results (i.e., DNA damage, cell stress signaling, pro-inflammatory p65 signaling) was validated by immunohistochemistry (Figure 13D).

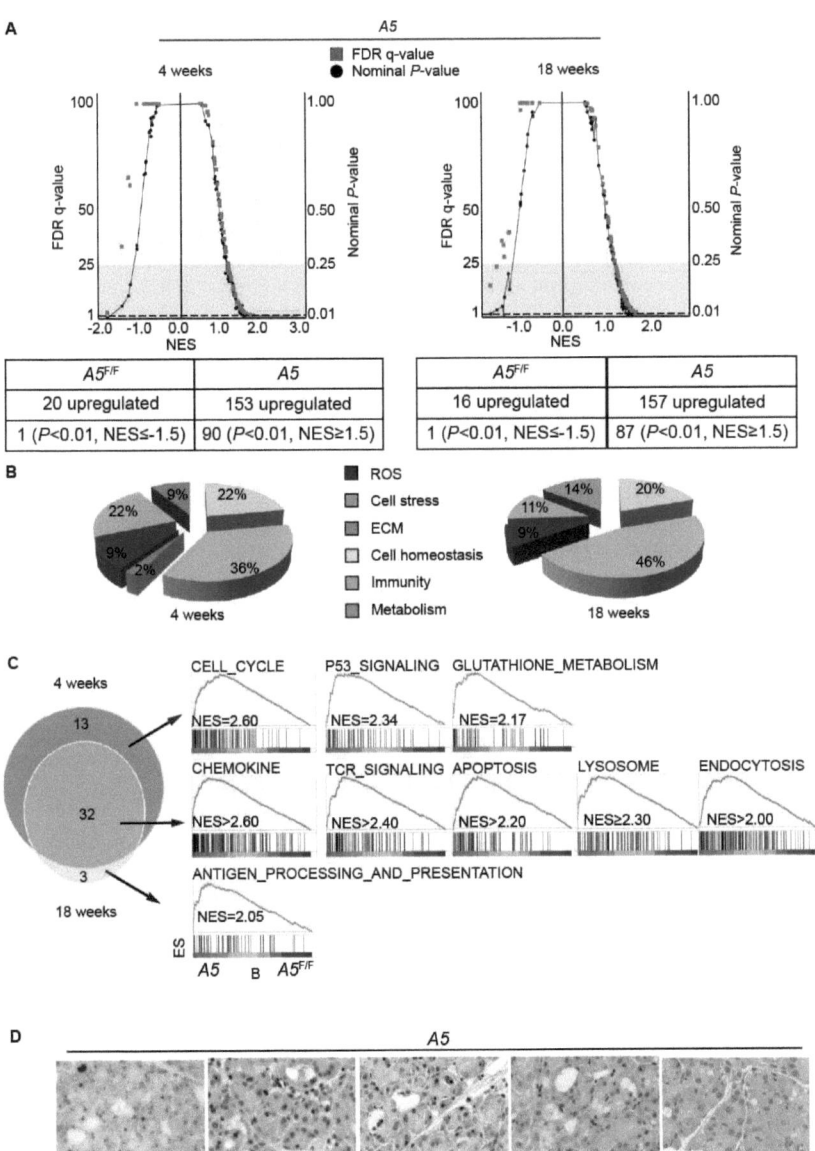

Figure 13: Whole-genome transcriptomics in A5 pancreata reveal increased ROS, immune signaling and disturbed cell homeostasis. (**A**) Normalized enrichment score (=NES) versus significance (nominal P-values, black circles, and false discovery rate (FDR) q-values, red quadrants) plots illustrating gene sets enriched in either A5 (n=3 per age group) or $A5^{F/F}$ (n=2) male pancreata at 4 (left) and 18 (right) weeks of age; gene sets were identified by GSEA using 173 KEGG pathway gene sets; 153 and 157 were upregulated in pancreata from 4- and 18-week old A5 mice (NES≥0.5) compared to 20 and 16 in pancreata from 4- and 18-week old control mice (NES≤-0.5) respectively; of those 90 and 87 were significantly enriched in pancreata from 4- and 18-week old A5 mice (NES≥1.5, nominal P-value<0.01), respectively compared to 1 in either pancreata from 4- and 18-week old control mice (NES≤-1.5, nominal P-value<0.01); the enriched pathways are localized beneath the dotted line in diagrams for 4- and 18-week old mice. (**B**) Classification of highly enriched gene sets into categories, based on the KEGG-pathway description for pancreatic tissue from 4- (left) and 18-week old (right) male A5 mice; NES≥2.0 and nominal P-value<0.001 were used to determine highly significant enrichment (ROS=reactive oxygen species, ECM=extracellular matrix) (see also Figure 14). (**C, left**) Venn diagram illustrating overlapping pathways highly enriched in pancreatic tissue of 4- and 18-week old male A5 mice (NES≥2.0, nominal P-value<0.001); dark gray, medium and light gray correspond to pathways enriched in pancreatic tissue from only 4-, both 4- and 18-, and only 18-week old mice, respectively (13, 32, and 3 pathways; see also Figure 14); (**C, right**) enrichment plots with examples of highly upregulated pathways (ES=enrichment score, TCR=T cell receptor; illustrations for common pathways in the middle originate from pancreata from 4-week old mice). (**D**) Immunohistochemical analyses for γH2Ax, phopsho-ERK, phopsho-p38, phospho-cJun and phospho-p65 in pancreata from 4-week old A5 mice; scale bars equal 50 μm.

4 weeks	4 and 18 weeks	18 weeks
NOD_LIKE_RECEPTOR_SIGNALING	B_CELL_RECEPTOR_SIGNALING	ANTIGEN_PROCESSING_AND_PRESENTATION
CELL_CYCLE	CHEMOKINE_RECEPTOR_SIGNALING	NEUROTROPHIN_SIGNALING
p53_SIGNALING	T_CELL_RECEPTOR_SIGNALING	ADHERENS_JUNCTION
PROSTATE_CANCER	NATURAL_KILLER_CELL_MEDIATED_CYTOTOXICITY	
PANCREATIC_CANCER	FC_GAMMA_R_MEDIATED_PHAGOCYTOSIS	
SPLICEOSOME	LEUKOCYTE_TRANSENDOTHELIAL_MIGRATION	
MISMATCH_REPAIR	HEMATOPOIETIC_CELL_LINEAGE	
RNA_DEGRADATION	TOLL_LIKE_RECEPTOR_SIGNALING	
EPITHELIAL_CELL_SIGNALING_IN_H_PYLORI_INFECTION	LEISHMANIA_INFECTION	
HOMOLOGOUS_RECOMBINATION	COMPLEMENT_AND_COAGULATION_CASCADE	
VEGF_SIGNALING	PRIMARY_IMMUNODEFICIENCY	
GLUTATHIONE_METABOLISM	PATHOGENIC_ESCHERICHIA_COLI_INFECTION	
AMINO_SUGAR_AND_NUCLEOTIDE_SUGAR_METABOLISM	CYTOKINE_CYTOKINE_RECEPTOR_INTERACTION	
	FC_EPSILON_RI_SIGNALING	
	INTESTINAL_IMMUNE_NETWORK_FOR_IGA_PRODUCTION	
	SMALL_CELL_LUNG_CANCER	
	DNA_REPLICATION	
	APOPTOSIS	
	CHRONIC_MYELOID_LEUKEMIA	
	COLORECTAL_CANCER	
	PATHWAYS_IN_CANCER	
	CELL_ADHESION_MOLECULES_CAMS	
	ECM_RECEPTOR_INTERACTION	
	FOCAL_ADHESION	
	REGULATION_OF_ACTIN_CYTOSKELETON	
	LYSOSOME	
	CYTOSOLIC_DNA_SENSING	
	ENDOCYTOSIS	
	VIRAL_MYOCARDITIS	
	SYSTEMIC_LUPUS_ERYTHEMATOSUS	
	METABOLISM_OF_XENOBIOTICS_BY_CYTOCHROME_P450	
	DRUG_METABOLISM_CYTOCHROME_P450	

Figure 14. KEGG pathway classification. Table illustrating KEGG-pathways highly enriched in 4- (left), both 4- and 18- (middle), and 18-week old (right) *A5* mice (NES≥2.0, nominal *P*-value<0.001); colors represent colors used for KEGG-pathway classification in Figure 13B and 13C.

For metabolomic analysis 4-week old male mice were selected. Multiple changes were detected in pathways associated with energy production (e.g., glycolysis, TCA cycle), anabolism (e.g., pentose phosphate pathway, reductive TCA cycle, lipid synthesis, amino acid synthesis), and ROS-detoxification (e.g., GSH cycle, peroxisome) (Figure 15). Interestingly, glutamate was found to feed into most of the upregulated pathways (Figure 15). Of those pathways identified, GSH and reductive TCA cycle were especially important since metabolomic and transcriptomic analysis suggested ROS accumulation and reduced fatty acid levels, indicating glutamate deficiency (Figure 15).

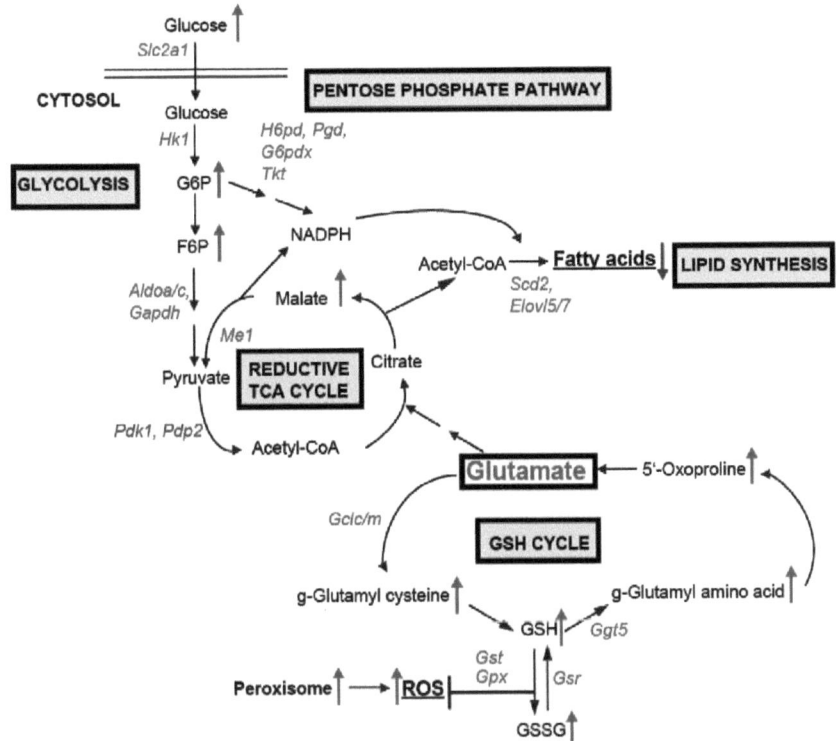

Figure 15: Combined transcriptomics and non-targeted metabolomics in A5 pancreata reveal alterations in glutamate-associated metabolic pathways.
Illustration of metabolic pathways upregulated in pancreatic tissue from 4-week old male A5 mice (yellow boxes) as identified by non-targeted metabolomics ($n=6$); up-/downregulated metabolites in A5 mice are indicated with red/blue arrows, respectively; enzymes involved in the respective pathways and identified by transcriptomics are shown with red/blue for up-/downregulation, respectively; glutamate is boxed and highlighted in green; ROS and fatty acids showing an increase and a decrease, respectively are underlined.

Abbreviations: Slc2a1=solute carrier family 2 (facilitated glucose transporter), member 1; Hk1=Hexokinase 1; H6pd=hexose-6-phosphate dehydrogenase; G6pdx=glucose-6-phosphate dehydrogenase X-linked; Pgd=phosphogluconate dehydrogenase; Tkt=transketolase; Aldoa=aldolase A; Aldoc=aldolase C; Gapdh=glyceraldehyde-3-phosphate dehydrogenase; Pdk1=pyruvate dehydrogenase kinase, isoenzyme 1; Pdp2=pyruvate dehyrogenase phosphatase catalytic subunit 2; Me1=malic enzyme 1, NADP(+)-dependent, cytosolic; Scd2=stearoyl-Coenzyme A desaturase 2; Elovl5=ELOVL family member 5, (for elongation of long chain fatty acids); Elovl7= ELOVL family member 7 (for elongation of long chain fatty acids); Gclc=glutamate-cysteine ligase, catalytic subunit; Gclm=glutamate-cysteine ligase, modifier subunit; Gpx=glutathione peroxidase; Gst=glutathione S-transferase; Gsr=glutathione reductase; Ggt5=gamma-glutamyltransferase 5;
G6P=glucose-6-phophsate; F6P=fructose-6-phosphate; CoA=Co-enzyme A; NADPH=nicotinamide adenine dinucleotide phosphate; GSH=glutathione; GSSG=glutathione disulfide; ROS=reactive oxygen species; TCA=tricarboxylic acid.

In summary, transcriptomics analysis provided additional evidence for an involvement of Atg5-dependent autophagy in CP. Indeed, with increasing age *A5* mice showed significant upregulation of ECM and immunity-related processes, indicative of increased fibrosis and inflammation. Both fibrosis and inflammation are crucially involved in pathology of CP. Combined transcriptomic and metabolomic analyses further uncovered a novel mechanism potentially underlying the *A5* pancreatic phenotype: ROS accumulation and elevated cell stress may lead to high glutamate requirements, ultimately resulting in glutamate deficiency.

5.2.5 ER stress, ROS and mitochondrial damage in *A5* mice

Both transcriptomics and metabolomics emphasized the importance of ROS in dictating pancreatic damage in *A5* mice. Indeed, ROS were directly (Figure 16A) and indirectly detected by a greatly enhanced Nrf1/Nrf2-dependent antioxidant gene expression (Figure 16B). Transcription of *Sqstm1*, coding for the autophagy substrate p62 and regulated by oxidative stress, was also enhanced in pancreata from *A5* mice (Figure 16C).

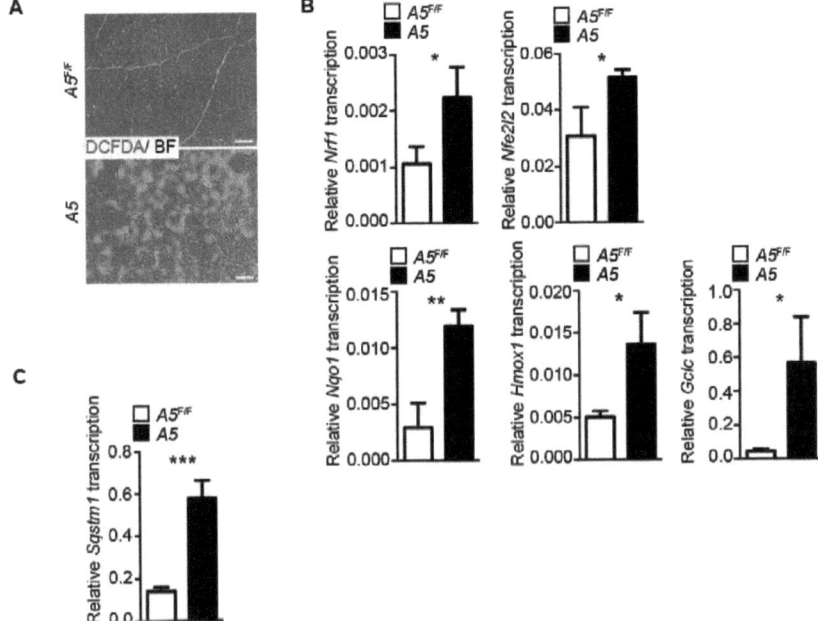

Figure 16. ROS accumulation and increased ROS-associated signaling in pancreata of A5 mice. (A) DCFDA-mediated fluorescent detection of reactive oxygen species (ROS) against bright field (BF) illumination in pancreatic acinar cells of 4-week old A5 and A5$^{F/F}$ mice; scale bar equals 50 μm. (B) Relative transcription of Nrf1, Nfe2l2, Nqo1, Hmox1, Gclc, and (C) Sqstm1 in whole pancreata from 4-week A5 mice (black bars) compared to controls (open bars); data are normalized to Cyclophilin; means±SD, (n=3), *P<0.05, **P<0.01, ***P<0.001.

It is known that autophagy regulates multiple aspects of cellular homeostasis ranging from metabolite production to intracellular organelle recycling[5]. In order to scrutinize the exact cellular changes leading to ROS-accumulation, electron microscopy was performed. Evidently, vacuolar structures found in acinar cells corresponded to greatly dilated ER cisternae (Figure 17A). ER-expansion is regulated by the unfolded protein response (UPR)[46]. UPR is activated upon ER stress conditions and may act to either restore ER homoeostasis (adaptive phase) or to induce apoptosis (apoptotic phase). Intensity and duration of cellular stress regulate switching between adaptive and apoptotic phase. Transcriptional analysis of pancreatic lysates from A5 mice revealed specific upregulation of apoptotic phase (*Atf3, Hspa5, Ddit3, Ppp1r15a, sXbp1*) but not adaptive phase (*Edem1, Dnajc3, P4hb*) effectors (Figure 17B and 17C). However, polyubiquitinated proteins, as a measure of unfolded protein accumulation could not be detected in *A5* pancreas at all time-points analyzed (Figure 17D). Damaged mitochondria were found in all acinar cells (Figure 17A). CREB is a known master regulator of mitochondrial biogenesis, influencing for example mitochondrial respiratory chain protein expression[47]. In *A5* pancreatic lysates pCREB/CREB-protein (Figure 17E) was found reduced, indicating disturbed mitochondrial biogenesis. Peroxisomes and lysosomes were also affected, since expression of PMP70, a peroxisomal marker, and Lamp2, a lysosomal marker, increased and decreased, respectively (Figure 17E).

A
A5
ER stress
Mitochondria
B
A5F/F
A5
Relative Atf3 transcription
0.008
0.006
0.004
0.002
0.000
*
Relative Hspa5 transcription
0.15
0.10
0.05
0.00
Relative Ddit3 transcription
***
Relative Ppp1r15a transcription
0.08
0.06
0.04
0.02
*
Relative Edem1 transcription
0.8
0.6
0.4
0.2
0.0
Relative Dnajc3 transcription
Relative P4hb transcription
3
2
1
0
C
A5F/F
A5
Xbp1u
Xbp1s
Cyclophilin
D
Ubi
100
75
50
37
25
β-actin
4
4
9
18
weeks
E
pCREB
CREB
PMP70
Lamp2
ERK12

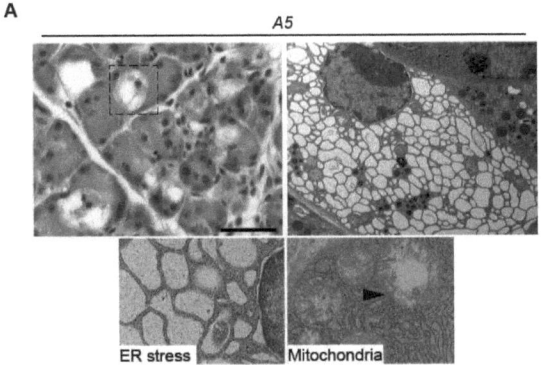

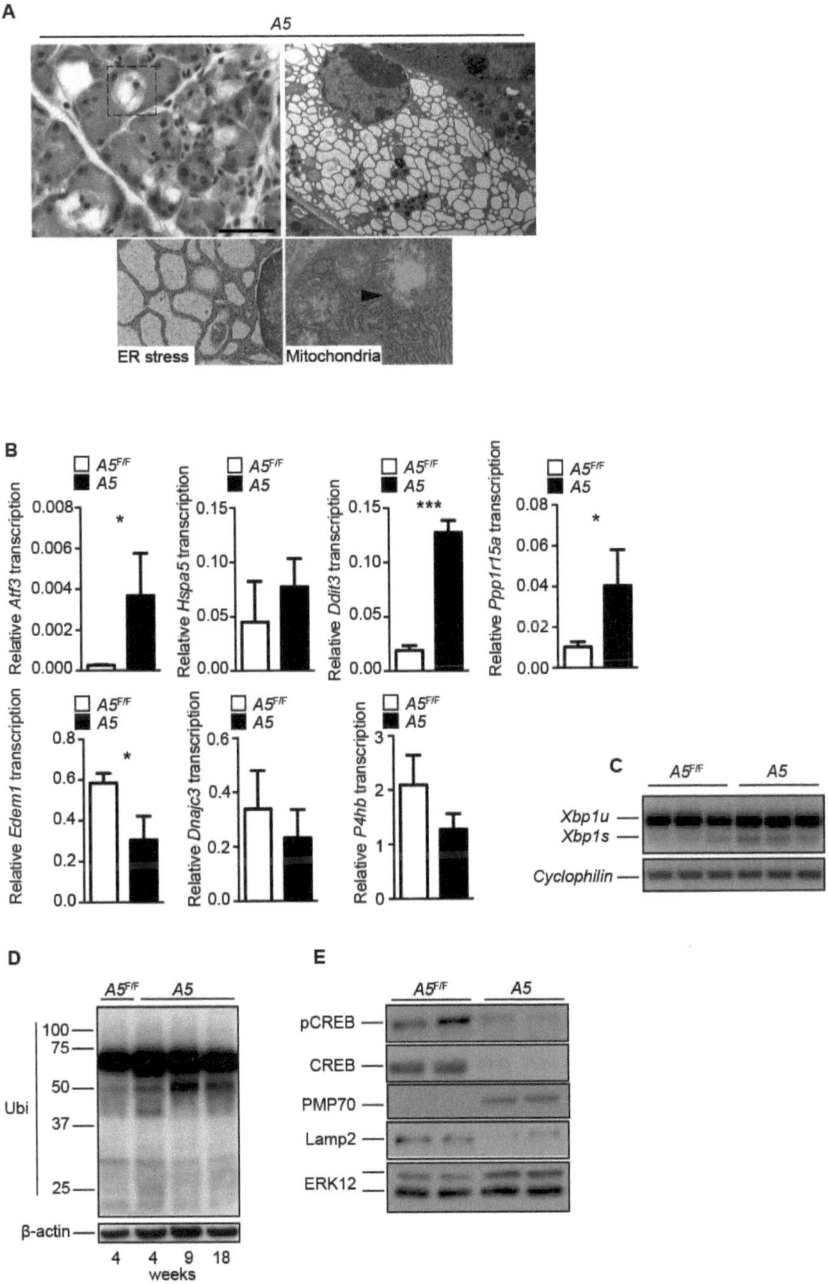

Figure 17. Disturbed organelle homeostasis in A5 pancreata. (A) H&E staining (top left, scale bar equals 50 μm) and ultrastructural overview (top right, 2000x) of pancreatic tissue from a 4-week old A5 mouse illustrate an example of stressed acinar cells (boxed area, left); (bottom from left to right) electron microscopy analysis (42000x) showing dilated endoplasmic reticulum (ER) cisternae as well as mitochondrial damage (arrowhead) in pancreatic acinar cells of 4-week old A5 mice. **(B)** Relative transcription of *Atf3*, *Hspa5*, *Ddit3*, *Ppp1r15a*, *Edem1*, *Dnajc3*, and *P4hb* in whole pancreata from 4-week old A5 mice (black bars) compared to controls (open bars); data are normalized to *Cyclophilin*; means±SD, (*n*=3), *$P<0.05$, ***$P<0.001$. **(C)** Detection of unspliced (*Xbp1u*) and spliced (*Xbp1s*) *Xbp1* mRNA in whole pancreatic homogenates from 4-week old A5 mice and controls by RT-PCR and agarose gel electrophoresis; *Cyclophilin* was used as an endogenous control. **(D)** Western blot mediated detection of polyubiquitinated proteins in pancreatic lysates from 4/9/18-week old A5 mice compared to controls; β-actin was used as loading control. **(E)** Western blot analysis of pCREB, CREB, PMP70, and Lamp2 in pancreatic lysates from 4-week old A5 mice compared to controls; ERK1 and 2 were used as loading controls.

Next, mitochondrial morphology and function were further scrutinized. Cardiolipin (CL) is found almost only in the mitochondrial membrane system and is required for maintenance of mitochondrial structure and function[48]. Lipidomics revealed a significantly reduced total CL and $(18:2)_4$-CL, the main pancreatic CL species, in pancreatic tissue from A5 mice (Figure 18A). At the same time, oxidation of $(C18:2)_4$-CL was increased (Figure 18A). Distribution of mitochondrial protein glutamate dehydrogenase activity (GLDH) into subcellular fractions provided a further measure of mitochondrial integrity. A5 mice displayed a more heterogeneous distribution in GLDH-activity and therefore mitochondrial density (Figure 18B). Peak GLDH-activity was also significantly reduced compared to wildtype controls (Figure 18B). Finally, activity of respiratory complex II (C II) and IV (C IV) was lower in isolated pancreatic mitochondria of A5 mice (Figure 18C).

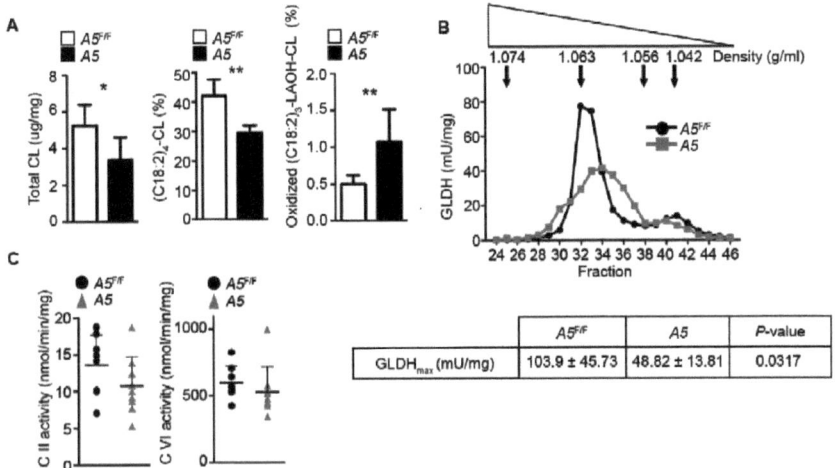

Figure 18. Compromised mitochondrial lipid composition and function in pancreas from A5 mice. (A) Quantification of total cardiolipin (total CL, μg/mg protein, left), (C18:2)$_4$-CL (in % total CL, middle) and oxidized (C18:2)$_3$-monohydroxylinoleic acid-CL (oxidized (C18:2)$_3$-LAOH-CL, in % of oxidized plus non oxidized (C18:2)$_4$-CL, right) in pancreata from 4-week old $A5^{F/F}$ (open bar) and A5 (black bar) mice by lipidomics; means±SD, (n≥7), *P<0.05, **P<0.01. (B) Mean glutamate dehydrogenase activity (GLDH, mU/mg protein) distribution into density fractions separated through density gradient centrifugation as a measure of mitochondrial integrity in pancreatic extracts from 4-week old male $A5^{F/F}$ (black line, black circle) and A5 (red line, red square) mice; the diagram illustrates the mean GLDH activity in fractions 24 to 46 with decreasing density (g/ml); table contains means±SD (n≥4) with *P<0.05 for peak GLDH (GLDHmax, mU/mg protein). (C) Quantification of respiratory complex II (C II) and IV (C IV) activity (nmol/min/mg) in mitochondrial extracts from 4-week old $A5^{F/F}$ (black circle) and A5 (red triangle) pancreata; means±SD, (n≥8).

Thus, pancreas-specific autophagy deficiency resulted in elevated ROS-levels, terminal ER stress, mitochondrial damage, accumulation of peroxisomes and alterations in lysosomes. Together, these defects led to acinar cell stress and subsequent apoptosis and/or necrosis, ultimately causing pancreatic organ damage.

5.3 Role of p53 and p62 in pancreas-specific autophagy deficiency

As previously demonstrated, p62 protein and mRNA levels were increased in *A5* mice (Figure 6 and 16C). Immunohistochemistry uncovered accumulation of p62 in intracellular aggregates of intact and stressed acinar cells (Figure 19A). The interaction of p62/Nrf2 and the consequences of continuous Nrf2-signaling upon autophagy deficiency were already described in the introduction. Interestingly, Nqo1, a downstream target of Nrf2, has been shown to stabilize p53 by inhibiting 20S proteasome-dependent degradation of p53[49]. Since p53 is a prominent effector of apoptosis/necrosis acting at the level of mitochondria[50], the p62/Nqo1/p53 pathway was analyzed in autophagy-deficient pancreas. *A5* mice displayed enhanced Nrf2-dependent gene transcription (Figure 16B) and increased Nqo1 protein expression (Figure 19A). Moreover, p53 expression was greatly enhanced along with p53-dependent gene expression (*Trp53, Cdkn1a, Bax, Bak1*) (Figure 19A and 19B).

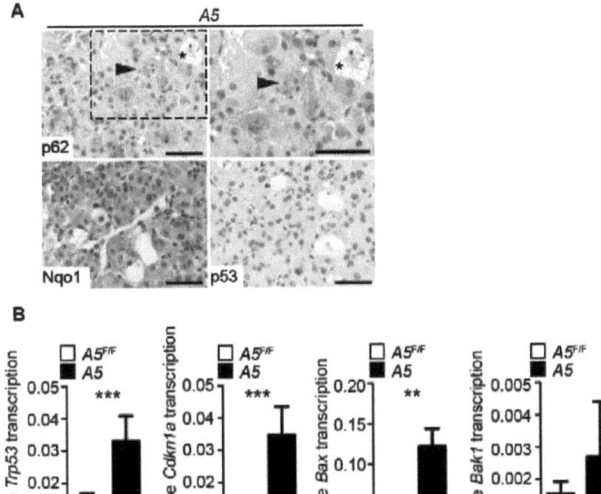

Figure 19. Increased p62/Nqo1/p53 expression and signaling in pancreata from A5 mice. (A) Immunohistochemical analyses for p62, Nqo1, and p53 expression in pancreatic tissue from 4-week old A5 mice; arrowhead and asterisk indicate p62 protein accumulation in cytoplasmic granula of intact acinar cells and acinar cells with severe ER stress respectively; the box outlines area magnified on the right: scale bars equal 50 µm. (B) Relative transcription of *Trp53*, *Cdkn1a*, *Bax*, and *Bak1* in whole pancreata from 4-week old A5 mice (black bars) compared to controls (open bars); data are normalized to *Cyclophilin*; means±SD, (n≥3), **$P<0.01$, ***$P<0.001$.

To scrutinize the importance of p53 and p62 in mediating pancreatic damage upon autophagy deficiency, *Atg5;Trp53* (termed *A5;p53*) as well as *Atg5;Sqstm1* (termed *A5;p62*) double deficient mice were generated. Surprisingly, both *A5;p53* and *A5;p62* mice lacked formation of intracellular vacuoles (Figure 20A). Moreover, mitochondrial morphology appeared normal (Figure 20B) and ROS-production was reduced (Figure 20C), supporting alleviation of oxidative, ER and mitochondrial stress. pCREB-levels were also increased in both *A5;p53* and *A5;p62* mice, reaching the expression level detected in wildtype controls (Figure 20D). Furthermore, quantification of BrdU and cleaved caspase 3, revealed reduced pancreatic acinar cell proliferation and apoptosis in both *A5;p53* and *A5;p62* mice (Figure 20E).

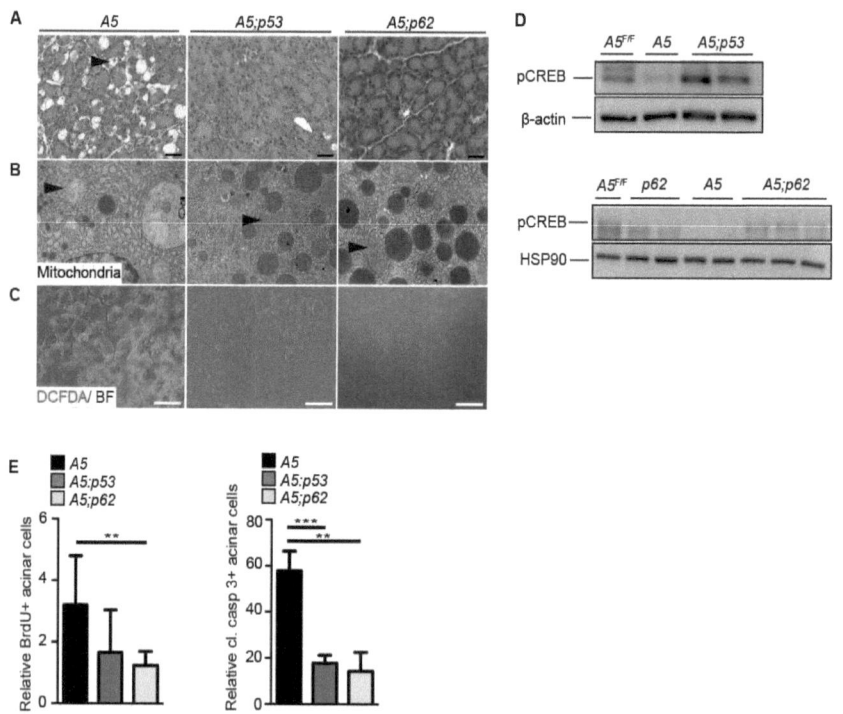

Figure 20. Reduced acinar cell stress, mitochondrial damage, and ROS accumulation in pancreata of A5;p53 and A5;p62 double deficient mice. (**A**) H&E-staining of pancreatic tissue from 4-week old mice with pancreas-specific deletion of either Atg5 and Trp53 (A5;p53, middle) or Atg5 and Sqstm1 (A5;p62, right) compared to age matched A5 controls (left); arrowhead indicates stressed acinar cells; scale bars equal 50 μm. (**B**) Electron microscopic images of acinar cells from 4-week old A5, A5;p53, and A5;p62 mice (13.000x) illustrating mitochondrial morphology (arrowhead). (**C**) DCFDA against bright field (BF) staining of pancreatic tissue sections from 4-week old A5, A5;p53, and A5;p62 mice; scale bars equal 50 μm. (**D**) Detection of pCREB in whole pancreatic lysates from 4-week old $A5^{F/F}$, A5 single deficient, and A5;p53 double deficient mice (top) as well as $A5^{F/F}$, p62, A5 single deficient, and A5;p62 double deficient mice (bottom), by western blot analysis; β-actin and HSP90 were used as loading controls. (**E**) Quantification of BrdU (left) and cleaved caspase 3 (right) positive acinar cells per high power field in pancreatic tissue from 4-week old A5 (black bar), A5;p53 (medium gray bar), and A5;p62 (light gray bar) mice relative to $A5^{F/F}$ mice; means±SD (n≥3), **P<0.01, ***P<0.001.

Thus, the results presented herein validated the importance of p62/Nqo1/p53 in mediating the pancreas-specific autophagy deficient phenotype. Indeed, p62 and p53 not only accumulated in autophagy deficient pancreata, but were also required for development of acinar cell stress further exacerbating necrosis/apoptosis in A5 mice.

5.4 Influence of gender

Surprisingly, separate monitoring of male and female A5 mice revealed a striking gender-mediated effect on pancreatic regeneration. At 4 weeks of age pancreata from male and female mice were macroscopically and histologically indistinguishable from each other, showing a similar degree of acinar cell vacuolization (Figure 21A and 21B). At older time-points however, notable differences appeared. While pancreatic degeneration (Figure 21A), acinar cell vacuolization, hypertrophic acinar cells, and persisting ductal-structures were evident in male *A5* mice (Figure 21B), females displayed almost normal pancreatic morphology (Figure 21A and 21B). In fact, only a few infiltrating cells could be detected (Figure 21B). Accordingly, pancreas to body weight was significantly elevated in female compared to male *A5* mice (Figure 21C). ROS (Figure 21D), apoptosis, fibrosis, and inflammation were increased in male *A5* mice; proliferation however was similar in both sexes, indicating ongoing regeneration in female pancreata (Figure 21E). The used pancreas-specific promoter Ptf1a targets not only the exocrine but also endocrine β-cells. Consequently, significant differences could be found in islet cell morphology, with male *A5* mice exhibiting almost complete islet disintegration (Figure 21E). Islet cell function was also compromised in male *A5* mice (Figure 21F). Specifically, 18-week old *A5* males had approximately double the amount of baseline serum glucose compared to wildtype controls, while female *A5* mice maintained normal baseline serum glucose levels (Figure 21F).

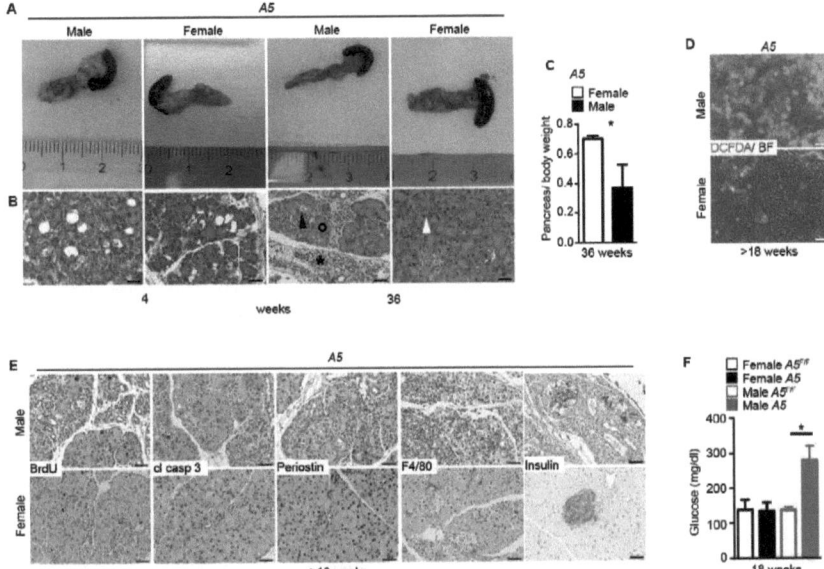

Figure 21. Pancreatic regeneration in A5 mice is gender dependent. (A) Macroscopic and (B) microscopic (H&E) pancreatic phenotype in male and female A5 mice at 4 and 36 weeks of age; black arrowhead, circle, asterisk, and white arrowhead indicate vacuolization, hypertrophic acinar cells, duct-like structures, and infiltrating cells, respectively; scale bars equal 50 µm. (C) Pancreas/body weight in female (open bar) and male (black bar) 36-week old A5 mice; means±SD, ($n \geq 3$), *$P<0.05$. (D) Fluorescent detection of ROS-generation by DCFDA against bright field (BF) illumination in pancreata from > 18-week old male and female A5 mice; scale bar equals 50 µm. (E) Immunohistochemical examination of BrdU, cleaved caspase 3, periostin, F4/80, and insulin in pancreata from male (top) and female (bottom) A5 mice at > 18 weeks of age; scale bars equal 50 µm. (F) Random serum glucose concentration (mg/dl) in 18-week old male (red bar) and female (black bar) A5 mice compared to the respective $A5^{F/F}$ controls (males, open red bar and females, open black bar); means±SD, ($n \geq 3$), *$P<0.05$.

Thus, in contrast to males, females could compensate loss of acinar cells, regenerating exocrine pancreatic tissue and maintaining endocrine pancreatic function.

5.5 Induction of acute pancreatitis

Impaired pancreatic autophagy significantly elevated acinar cell stress leading to pancreatic organ damage and loss of regeneration in male mice. In order to elucidate if impaired autophagy also affects resistance to experimental AP, A5 mice were subjected to hourly, i.p. cerulein injections (Figure 22A).

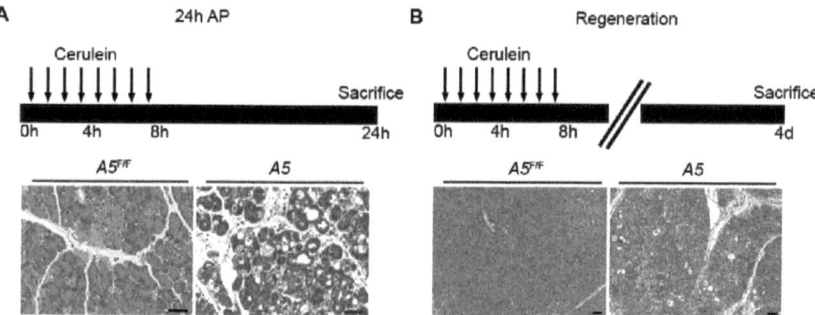

Figure 22. Pancreatic autophagy protects from acute pancreatitis and facilitates regeneration. (A) Induction of 24 h acute pancreatitis (AP) in A5 and $A5^{F/F}$ mice; (top) experimental scheme illustrating hourly, intraperitoneal cerulein injection starting from 0 h and ending at 8 h, including a total of 8 injections; mice were sacrificed 24 h after the first injection; (bottom) microscopic (H&E) examination of A5 and $A5^{F/F}$ mice; scale bars equal 50 μm. (B) Pancreatic regeneration after AP induction; (top) experimental scheme illustrating AP induction as described under (A); mice were sacrificed 4 days after first injection; (bottom) microscopic (H&E) examination of A5 and $A5^{F/F}$ mice; scale bars equal 50 μm.

A5 mice exhibited significantly more acinar cell vacuolization compared to control mice (Figure 22A). Inflammatory cell infiltration was also increased (Figure 22A). Moreover, pancreatic regeneration after AP induction was greatly compromised; indeed acinar cell vacuolization and ductal structures were increasingly evident in the pancreas of A5 mice 4 days after AP, compared to the pancreas of control mice (Figure 22B).

In support of an increased AP severity after autophagy deficiency, serum activities of amylase and lipase were also elevated at baseline and 4 h after AP-induction in A5 mice compared to wildtype mice (Figure 23).

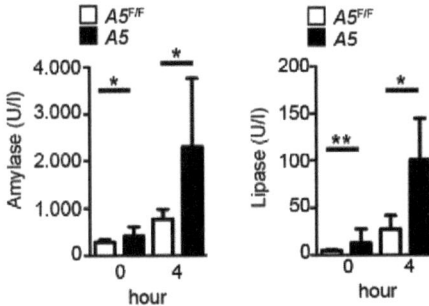

Figure 23. Pancreatic autophagy reduces severity of acute pancreatitis. Serum amylase (left) and lipase (right) activities (U/l) in A5 (black bar) compared to $A5^{F/F}$ (open bar) 0 (n=10 per group) and 4 (n=4 per group) hours after AP induction, as described in Figure 22A; means±SD, *P<0.05, **P<0.01.

Thus, impaired pancreatic autophagy also compromised resistance of acinar cells to cerulein-induced cell stress and pancreatic regeneration.

5.6 Influence of diet

In order to obtain definite evidence for the detrimental effect of ROS accumulation and reduced availability of anabolic substrates in autophagy-deficient pancreata, male A5 mice were treated with a specific dietary formulation. A 25% palm oil diet (POD) was chosen and compared to standard diet (SD) (Table 12).

Table 12: Dietary analysis of POD compared to SD. Percentages refer to the mass % in the diet; metabolizable energy (ME, MJ/kg); calories from protein, fat, and carbohydrates (kJ%) are calculated using Atwater factors; SD=Standard Diet, POD=Palm Oil Diet.

Component	SD	POD
ME	12.5 MJ/kg	19.7 MJ/kg
Fat	5.1% (13 kJ%)	25.1% (48 kJ%)
Protein	22.8 (27 kJ%)	21.2% (18 kJ%)
Carbohydrates	33.3% (60 kJ%)	26.7% (34%)
Palmitic acid (C16:0)	0.5%	9.18%
Arachidic acid (C20:0)	0.02%	0.1%
Oleic acid (C18:1)	0.9%	9.19%
Linoleic acid (C18:2)	2.1%	4.67%
Amino acids	Similar	Similar
Vitamins	More Vit A	More Vit D3, E
Minerals/Trace elements	Similar	Similar

Palm oil is a rich source vitamin E with potent antioxidant capacities. Moreover, palm oil contains palmitic and oleic acid in a ratio of 1:1, providing optimal fatty acid combination[51,52]. Another set of mice was given drinking water supplemented with the antioxidant N-acetylcysteine (NAC). Dietary treatment started at 4 weeks of age and ended at 18 weeks of age (Figure 24A). After being fed POD, fat accumulation (Figure 24B) and significantly increased body weight were evident in wildtype but not *A5* mice (Figure 24C).

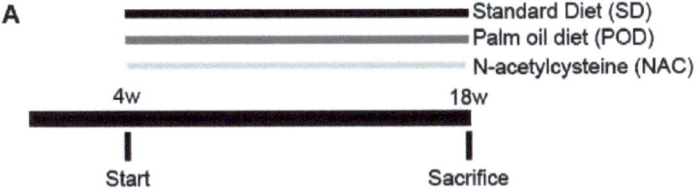
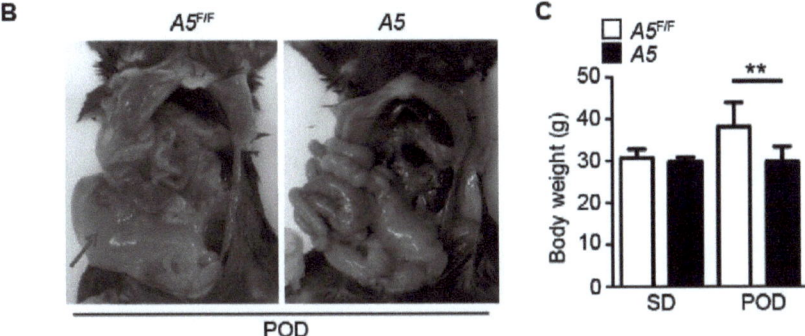

Figure 24. Dietary treatment of male A5 mice and effects on body weight. (A) Schematic illustrating feeding or treatment of male $A5^{F/F}$ and A5 mice with standard diet (SD, black bar), palm oil diet (POD, medium grey bar), or N-acetylcysteine (NAC, light gray bar) for 14 weeks starting at 4 and ending at 18 weeks of age. (B) Picture illustrating accumulation of omental fat in $A5^{F/F}$ (red arrow), but not A5 mice fed POD. (C) Body weight (g) of 18-week old male $A5^{F/F}$ (open bar) and A5 (black bar) mice fed SD or POD; means±SD, ($n≥4$), **$P<0.01$.

Surprisingly, morphological comparison of A5 and $A5^{F/F}$ mice (Figure 25A and 25B) and quantification of relative acinar cell area (Figure 25C) revealed significant increases in POD-treated A5 mice. In addition POD significantly increased relative amylase and elastase transcription in A5 mice (Figure 25D and 25E). NAC-treatment also improved pancreatic structure, although some regenerative areas remained (Figure 25A, 25B and 25C).

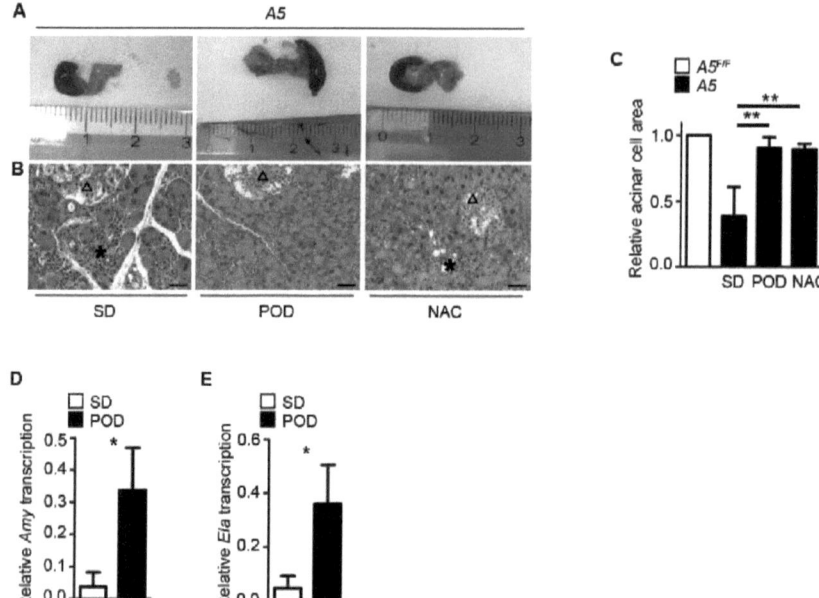

Figure 25. Rescue of CP phenotype after feeding A5 mice a diet rich in vitamin E and oleic acid or treatment with N-acetylcysteine. (A) Macroscopic and (B) microscopic (H&E) examination of POD-fed or NAC-treated A5 mice, compared to A5 mice fed with SD; asterisk and triangle indicate duct-like structures and islets, respectively; scale bars equal 50 μm. (C) Quantification of acinar to total pancreatic area (relative acinar cell area) in A5 (black bar) mice fed SD or POD or treated with NAC and compared to $A5^{F/F}$ (open bar) mice fed SD; means±SD, ($n≥3$), **$P<0.01$. (D) Relative transcription of Amylase (Amy) and (E) Elastase (Ela) in whole pancreata of 18-week old A5 mice after being fed SD (open bar) or POD (black bar); data are normalized to Cyclophilin and depicted in relation to $A5^{F/F}$ mice; means±SD, ($n≥3$), *$P<0.05$.

Moreover, POD was able to dramatically improve mitochondrial morphology, as examined by electron microscopy (Figure 26A), and mitochondrial lipid oxidation (Figure 26C) while significantly alleviating ROS accumulation (Figure 26B). NAC-treatment did not affect mitochondrial morphology (Figure 26A) but was able to reduce ROS-production, albeit at a lower degree compared to POD (Figure 26B). In addition, quantification of BrdU and cleaved caspase 3 demonstrated a reduction of positive acinar cells in *A5* mice fed POD compared to *A5* mice fed SD (Figure 26D and 26E). Finally, western blot was performed to detect alterations in autophagic signaling, acinar cell damage and intracellular organelle composition. While *A5* mice fed POD still displayed loss of Atg5-expression and LC3-lipidation, p62 accumulated to a lower degree compared to SD-fed *A5* mice (Figure 26F). In addition, POD reverted cleavage of CPA and expression of Lamp2, PMP70 and pCREB in *A5* mice compared to SD-fed *A5* mice (Figure 26F).

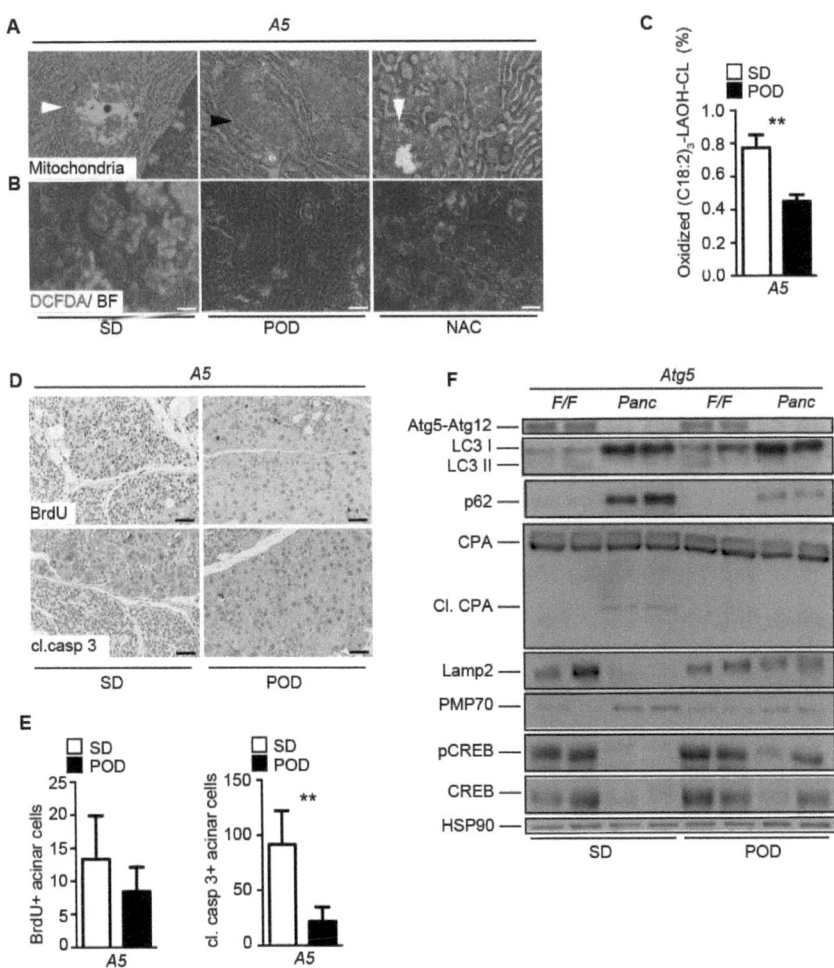

Figure 26. Rescue of mitochondrial morphology, ROS-accumulation and acinar cell proliferation/apoptosis and reversal of p62, cleaved CPA, Lamp2, PMP70 and pCREB expression in POD-fed A5 mice. (A) Electron microscopy (30,000x) of A5 mice fed with SD or POD or treated with NAC; white and black arrowheads indicate damaged and intact mitochondria, respectively. (B) DCFDA against bright field (BF) staining of pancreatic tissue sections from A5 mice fed SD or POD or treated with NAC; scale bars equal 50 µm. (C) Quantification of oxidized $(C18:2)_3$-monohydroxylinoleic acid-CL (oxidized $(C18:2)_3$-LAOH-CL, in % of oxidized plus non oxidized $(C18:2)_4$-CL) in pancreatic extracts from 4-week old A5 mice fed with SD (open bar) and 18-week old A5 mice fed with POD (black bar) based on lipidomics analysis; means±SD, (n=3), **P<0.01. (D) Immunohistochemical detection of proliferation (BrdU, top) and apoptosis (cleaved caspase 3, bottom) in 18-week old A5 mice fed SD or POD; scale bars equal 50 µm. (E) Quantification of BrdU (left) and cleaved caspase 3 (right) positive acinar cells per acinar cell area (µm^2) in 18-week old A5 mice fed SD (open bar) or POD (black bar) relative to $A5^{F/F}$; means±SD, (n≥3), **P<0.01. (F) Western blot analysis for Atg5, LC3 I/II, p62, CPA/cl. CPA, Lamp2, PMP70, pCREB, and CREB in pancreatic extracts from 4-week old $A5^{F/F}$ and A5 mice fed with SD and 18-week old $A5^{F/F}$ and A5 mice fed POD; HSP90 was used as loading control.

Of note, islets retained damaged architecture in A5 mice and were not affected by any treatment (Figure 27A). Indeed glycemic control as measured by baseline serum glucose (Figure 27B) and i.p. glucose injection (Figure 27C) was impaired in A5 compared to $A5^{F/F}$ mice after POD feeding.

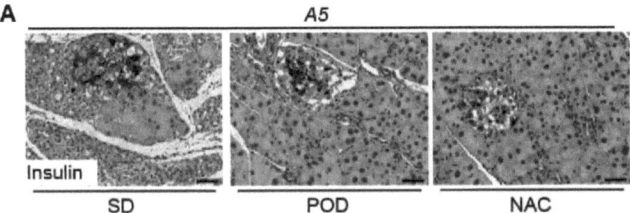

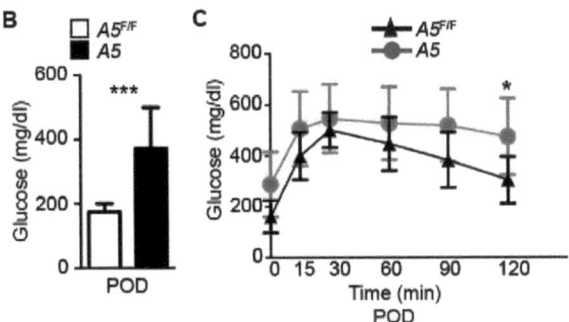

Figure 27. Morphology and function of the endocrine compartment in A5 mice is not altered by palm oil or NAC. (A) Immunohistochemical detection of insulin in pancreatic islets from 18-week old A5 mice after being fed SD or POD, or being treated with NAC; scale bars equal 50 μm. (B) Random serum glucose concentrations (mg/dl) in 18-week old male $A5^{F/F}$ (open bar) and A5 (black bar) mice fed POD; means±SD, (n≥8), ***P<0.001. (C) IPGTT (glucose mg/dl) in 18-week old POD-fed male $A5^{F/F}$ (black line, black triangle) and A5 (red line, red circle) mice; means±SD, (n≥8), *P<0.05.

Thus, antioxidants and essential fatty acids were able to rescue exocrine but not endocrine pancreatic phenotype in autophagy deficient pancreata.

5.7 Similarities with human chronic pancreatitis

To support the relevance of the A5-model for human CP, the pancreatic phenotype of CP patients was analyzed. A focus was placed on major signaling pathways identified in the previous experiments.

Similar to autophagy-deficient *A5* mice, acinar cell stress, metaplasia and ER stress were seen in CP-patients (Figure 28A and 28B). In addition, mitochondrial damage was evident (Figure 28B) along with significant reductions in total CL and $(C18:2)_4$-CL in pancreatic tissue from CP patients (Figure 28C). However, oxidation of $(C18:2)_4$-CL remained the same (Figure 28C).

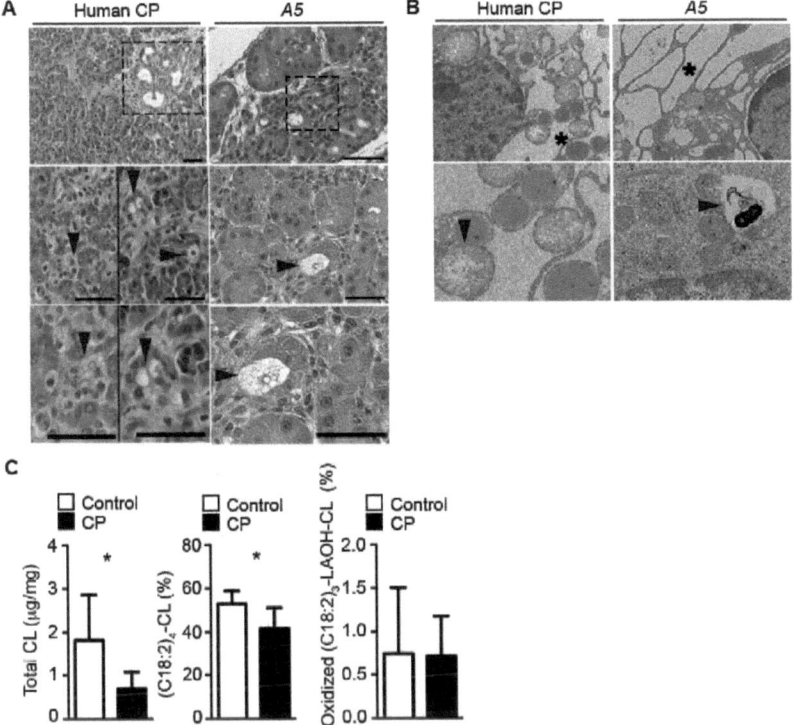

Figure 28. Similarities in histology and mitochondrial morphology between pancreatic tissue from A5 mice and human CP. (A) H&E staining of pancreatic tissue from human chronic pancreatitis (CP) patients (left) and 18-week old A5 mice (right); arrowheads indicate stressed acinar cells; duct-like structures are boxed; scale bars equal 50 μm. (B) Electron microscopy analysis of pancreatic acinar cells from human CP patients (left) and A5 mice (right) illustrating dilated ER cisternae (asterisk) and damaged mitochondria (arrowhead) (top 14,000x, bottom 34,000x). (C) Quantification of total cardiolipin (total CL, μg/mg protein, left), $(C18:2)_4$-CL (in % total CL, middle) and oxidized $(C18:2)_3$-monohydroxylinoleic acid-CL (oxidized $(C18:2)_3$-LAOH-CL, in % of oxidized plus non oxidized $(C18:2)_4$-CL, right) in pancreatic tissue from healthy human control (open bar) and human CP patients (black bar) by lipidomics; means±SD, (n=6), *$P<0.05$.

In addition to the morphological similarities, the proposed feed-forward loop of p62/Nqo1/p53 also appeared to be active in specimens from human CP patients. Indeed p62, Nqo1 and p53 could be found expressed in sequential pancreatic tissue sections from human CP patients (Figure 29).

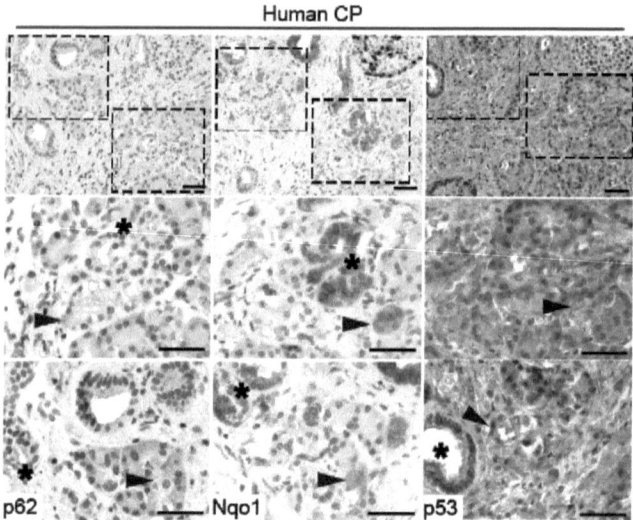

Figure 29. Induction of p62/Nqo1/p53 signaling in pancreatic tissue from human CP patients. Immunohistochemical detection of p62, Nqo1, and p53 in sequential pancreatic tissue sections from human CP patients; boxed areas in the top row are magnified in the middle and bottom rows; arrowheads indicate acinar cells and asterisks duct-like structures; scale bars equal 50 µm.

However, exon sequencing of *ATG5* in pancreatic tissue from human CP patients did not reveal any genetic alterations associated with CP (Table 13).

Table 13: *ATG5* exon sequencing in human CP patients. 267 CP patients and 241 healthy controls were evaluated for various *ATG5* variants.

Variant	CP (*n*=267)	Controls (*n*=241)	*P*-value
c.237-8A>G (hetero)	4/267 (1.5%)	5/241 (2.1%)	0.6
c.316-21gA	34/267 (12.7%)	40/241 (16.6%)	0.2
c.316-21AA	0/267 (0%)	1/241 (0.4%)	0.2
c.444G>A (p.K148K)	11/267 (4.1%)	6/241 (2.5%)	0.3
c.573+43CT	1/267 (0.4%)	0/241 (0%)	0.2
c.692-18gA	43/267 (16.1%)	43/241 (17.8%)	0.6
c.692-18AA	1/267 (0.4%)	2/241 (0.8%)	0.5

Thus, autophagic degradation appeared to be blocked in human CP, resulting in ER stress, mitochondrial damage, and p62/Nqo1/p53- accumulation. However, the lack of genetic alterations in *ATG5* exons in human CP implied that ATG5 indepent signaling mechanisms were influenced in human CP.

6 DISCUSSION

Autophagy is an important cellular homeostatic mechanism influencing physiology and pathophysiology of multiple tissue types[5]. The two main functions of autophagy include nutrient supply and alleviation of cell stress by organelle recycling and protein aggregate degradation[5]. Acinar cells of the exocrine pancreas synthesize, store, and secrete multiple enzymes and zymogens necessary for digestion and nutrient absorption. Consequently, acinar cells synthesize large quantities of protein that require effective homeostatic mechanisms and sufficient nutrient supply. Interestingly, levels of baseline and starvation induced autophagy are higher in the exocrine pancreas when compared to other organs ([24] and results shown here). As shown in this study and in others[24], autophagosome numbers are also increased after experimental AP. Autophagy has therefore been suggested to play an important homeostatic role in the exocrine pancreas. However, definite results are lacking. Also, inconsistencies have been reported, warranting further investigation (compare [40] and e.g. [53]).

The aim of this study was to shed light on the role of autophagy in pancreatic physiology and disease. Pancreatitis, both acute and chronic, is a complex disease affecting exocrine pancreatic morphology and function. The pathophysiological mechanism leading to pancreatitis has not been definitively elucidated and treatment options remain few, aiming mostly to alleviate disease symptoms[22,23]. Currently, there is no treatment for patients with CP and most patients remain symptomatic[23]. Variability in disease symptoms among patients further complicates the management of this disease[23]. Development of novel therapies requires accurate pre-clinical evaluation and therefore animal models that are able to recapitulate all stages and the variability of human pancreatitis are necessary[54]. In addition, clinical scenarios need to be simulated in experimental models[54]. AP is diagnosed at stages when necrosis and inflammation are at their peak[54]. Early diagnosis of CP is difficult as definitive evidence is usually lacking and CP can be mistaken for AP[23]. Laboratory studies analyze the impact of potential therapies usually prior to disease onset or during early stages of disease[54]. Thus, a more accurate treatment evaluation would be achieved in models of AP or CP, when applied during the peak of symptom development[54]. In the present study, mice deficient in pancreatic autophagy emerged as a novel model for human CP, mirroring multiple stages and symptoms of human CP, thus enabling development of new therapeutic strategies at later disease stages more relevant for the human condition.

6.1 Impaired pancreatic autophagy induces chronic atrophic CP

Tissue-specific impairments of autophagy have been described in multiple degenerative and inflammatory diseases and cancer types[5]. More specifically, autophagy has been associated with pancreatic diseases, including AP[24], CP[2,24], and pancreatic cancer[2]. However, no study has detailed the exact role of autophagy in exocrine pancreatic diseases.

In the present study, the role of pancreatic autophagy was analyzed by characterizing pancreas-specific *Atg5*-deficient mice. Interestingly, loss of pancreatic autophagy in mice recapitulated multiple traits of CP. Starting at 4 weeks of age, acinar cells exhibited evidence of increased cell stress, including cytosolic vacuolization, zymogen activation, and necrosis/apoptosis. Subsequent pancreatic tissue damage led to inflammation, organ enlargement and edema. The degree of acinar cell proliferation was also increased but was unable to compensate for the extensive tissue loss. Consequently, at later time-points (18 weeks of age) ineffective regeneration led to pancreatic atrophy, tissue remodeling, and fibrosis. Remaining acinar cells became hypertrophic, while lost acinar cells were replaced by structures expressing multiple ductal markers. On closer examination, ductal-like structures were indicative of acinar-to-ductal metaplasia, a mechanism known to be involved in pancreatic regeneration[55]. Nevertheless, while ductal structures retained loss of Atg5, they did not express embryonic or stem cell markers, indicating that pancreatic damage was not sufficient to trigger stem cell expansion[42], or that stem cells were also affected by autophagy deficiency[56]. Transcriptomic analysis further supported CP-development showing significant upregulation of fibrosis and inflammation-associated pathways. Simultaneously, A5 mice exhibited signs of cachexia, which represents a known consequence of CP[57]. Also, AP was further aggravated in autophagy-deficient mice, further supporting the important homeostatic role of Atg5-dependend autophagy in acinar cells with or without cellular stress. Of note, haploinsufficiency was not evident, as $Atg5^{F/-}$ mice did not display any morphological alterations.

Pancreatic autophagy seems to be required for maintenance of adult exocrine tissue. Indeed, newborn A5 mice (1 week of age) did not exhibit any morphological alterations of the pancreas. It is only after 4 weeks of age that evidence of acinar cell stress appeared. However, similar to results of a recent study, conditional deletion of Atg5 in acinar cells starting at 4 weeks of age did not disturb acinar cell homeostasis[40].

Thus, compared to existing CP models[58], loss of pancreatic autophagy in mice faithfully mirrored multiple features of human CP. Blockade of autophagic degradation has been associated with pancreatitis[24]. This study supported and expanded results from past studies characterizing in detail the effect of autophagy deficiency in the pancreas.

6.2 Defective mitochondria cause ROS accumulation and subsequent metabolic deficiencies in pancreata of *A5* mice

Oxidative stress plays an important role in pancreatitis[59-61]. Combined results from transcriptomics and metabolomics suggested persistent ROS-accumulation to have a central role in the *A5*-phenotype. Moreover, ROS were directly detected in pancreatic tissue of *A5* mice at all time-points analyzed. Multiple cellular sources of ROS exist, including mitochondria, peroxisomes, NADPH oxidases, P450 cytochrome, and the ER[62,63]. Detailed analysis of the pancreas of *A5* mice revealed extensive disruption of cellular homeostasis including ER dilatation, mitochondrial damage, peroxisome accumulation, and lysosomal alterations. Thus, autophagy deficient pancreatic acinar cells exhibited many potential ROS sources. Importantly, ER, mitochondria, peroxisomes, and to an extent also lysosomes are subject to autophagy-dependent homeostatic control[7]. Their accumulation therefore was a direct consequence of autophagy deficiency.

ER dilatation is indicative of ER stress and is induced by the UPR[46]. UPR stimulation may occur e.g., upon defective protein folding and protein accumulation, perturbation in calcium homeostasis, or alterations in redox metabolism[46]. In *A5* mice, alterations in redox metabolism were evident. Moreover, autophagy deficiency has been associated with accumulation of polyubiquitinated protein aggregates[5]. However ubiquitinated proteins, as a source of ER stress, were not detected in autophagy deficient pancreas. Thus, ROS seem to underlie UPR induction, especially as treatment of *A5* mice with the antioxidant NAC alleviated ER-stress. Importantly, ROS accumulation appeared to be so severe, that terminal ER stress was induced, driving pancreatic acinar cells to apoptosis.

Defective mitochondria are thought of as one of the main intracellular sources of ROS[62]. *A5* mice displayed several features of mitochondrial dysfunction, including morphological alterations, reduced total CL with simultaneous increases in oxidized CL, reduced pCREB/CREB, and decreased GLDHmax, respiratory complex II, and complex IV activity. Peroxisomal metabolism is also known to generate ROS[64] and in *A5* mice peroxisomes did accumulate. Thus, defective mitochondria and accumulating peroxisomes likely caused ROS accumulation in the pancreas of *A5* mice, subsequently driving acinar cells into apoptosis and/or necrosis. Interestingly, improved mitochondrial morphology and decreased accumulation of peroxisomes in pancreata of POD-treated *A5* mice were directly associated with reduced ROS-levels and cell damage, further supporting the central role of mitochondria and, to an extent, peroxisomes in the development of acinar cell stress.

Acinar cell metabolism was also affected by persistent ROS accumulation. Indeed, metabolomics revealed a highly upregulated glutathione metabolism, which is required for ROS detoxification. Interestingly, metabolomics also uncovered a high glutamate demand in *A5* pancreata. Glutamate is known to feed into multiple metabolic pathways[65] such as energy production (e.g., TCA cycle), anabolism (e.g., reductive TCA cycle, lipid synthesis, amino acid synthesis), and ROS-detoxification (e.g., GSH cycle). *A5* pancreata exhibited ROS accumulation and reduced fatty acid levels, indicative of insufficient detoxifying mechanisms and fatty acid synthesis, respectively. As glutamate is involved in both metabolic pathways, both alterations may be direct consequences of glutamate deficiency. Autophagy deficiency may also be directly involved in the observed metabolic deficiencies, as autophagy is known to supply cells with glutamine, a precursor of glutamate[66], as well as metabolic substrates such as fatty acids[5].

Thus, mitochondria and potentially peroxisomes were the main cellular sources of ROS in autophagy-deficient pancreas. ROS subsequently led to terminal ER stress-mediated apoptosis and/or necrosis and associated tissue damage. The high amounts of ROS also affected metabolism, as cells were required to upregulate their glutathione metabolism as well as fatty acid synthesis to reduce ROS and comply with increased membrane demands, respectively. Ultimately, this state led to increased glutamate use and thus resulted in glutamate deficiency.

6.3 The p62/Nrf2/Nqo1/p53 feed forward loop

The data presented herein uncovered a p62/Nrf2/Nqo1/p53-dependend feed-forward signaling pathway, mediating detrimental ROS-increases (Figure 30). The known interactions between p62/Nrf2 have been described above (3.1.4). Moreover, Nrf2-signaling is involved in p53 stabilization through Nqo1-induction, while p53-dependent p21 expression is involved in protecting Nrf2 from Keap1-mediated ubiquitination and degradation[49,67]. Thus, p62/Nrf2/p53 are able to interact, leading to diverse effects on cell survival, depending on the degree of cell stress[67].

In pancreatic tissue from A5 mice p62, Nqo1, and p53 protein as well as mRNA levels were significantly increased. Transcriptional activities of Nrf2 and p53 were also enhanced. P62-accumulation and persistent Nrf2-signaling have been detected in autophagy deficient liver, whereby Nrf2-activation was associated with liver injury[68] and liver adenomas[18]. Furthermore, simultaneous knockout of Sqstm1 or Nfe2l2 has been shown to ameliorate the phenotype of autophagy deficient liver cells and to abolish ubiquitin aggregate accumulation in autophagy deficient brain and liver cells[5,19]. P53, on the other hand, has not been shown to be directly involved in these phenotypes. However, p53 is known to mediate multiple pro-apoptotic/pro-necrotic effects at the level of mitochondria[50] and also to drive ROS production[69]. Interestingly, the genetic evidence obtained herein demonstrated that acinar cell stress depended on both *Sqstm1* and *Trp53*. Indeed, accumulation of defective mitochondria, ER stress, and ROS could be rescued with simultaneous *Sqstm1* or *Trp53* deletion in *A5* mice. Moreover, *Atg5* and *Sqstm1/Trp53* double-deficient acinar cells exhibited normal morphology and lacked intracellular vacuolization.

Thus, autophagy was required to regulate levels of important signaling effectors such as p62/Nrf2/Nqo1/p53. When autophagy was disabled, acinar cells accumulated p62 and to extent active Nrf2, Nqo1, and p53, ultimately exacerbating ROS-levels, necrosis/apoptosis and tissue damage.

6.4 The impact of gender and nutrition in regulating Atg5-dependent pathophysiology

Male gender is a known risk factor for CP-development. Moreover, nutritional aspects with respect to obesity, hypertriglyceridemia, and diabetes mellitus have been associated with AP[21]. Similarly, CP-development in *A5* mice was dependent on gender and nutrition. Chronic pancreatic tissue damage and degeneration was evident in male *A5* mice only. Additionally, feeding male *A5* mice with a combination of beneficial fatty acids and antioxidants was able to restore pancreatic regeneration.

It is known that antioxidative defense mechanisms vary among males and females. Studies have shown that male individuals generate higher amounts of ROS and show less effective mechanisms for elimination compared to females[70,71]. Moreover, autophagy has been shown to be under the regulation of hormones and ROS[70]. In this study female *A5* mice were able to effectively reduce ROS levels in pancreatic tissue compared to male *A5* mice. Endocrine pancreatic insufficiency as seen in male mice was also significantly reduced and islets exhibited normal morphology in female mice. Thus, this model suggested that autophagy was a crucial protective mechanism in the pancreas of males, whereas females appeared to possess sufficient alternative mechanisms for ROS-detoxification and tissue protection.

Taking into account the increased ROS-levels and demands for fatty acid anabolism due to pathologic ER-expansion and acinar cell turnover, supplementation of metabolic substrates was required for cells to cope with stress and regenerate pancreatic tissue. Accordingly, treatment of *A5* mice with antioxidants reduced ROS and protected from excessive damage. However, an even greater improvement was seen when mice were fed a palm oil rich-diet. Palm oil is known for its antioxidative capacities and beneficial fatty acids[51,52] and studies using tocotrienol, an important component of vitamin E in palm oil, have shown potent antifibrotic and antiinflammatory effects in rodent models of experimental pancreatitis [72,73] as well as antiproliferative effects in human pancreatic cancer cells[74]. Palm oil fed *A5* mice exhibited improved mitochondrial morphology, lipid composition and biogenesis, reduced ROS and digestive enzyme activation. Consequently, exocrine pancreatic tissue was completely regenerated. Of note, reduced p62 accumulation shown to occur in this study after palm oil feeding, further supports the role of p62 in mediating tissue damage. As opposed to the changes described in exocrine pancreatic tissue, endocrine pancreatic tissue was not affected by any treatment in *A5* mice.

In conclusion, ROS-accumulation determined CP-development in males, which could be prevented by antioxidants and beneficial fatty acids Thus, nutritional supplementation may be useful to block CP-progression during conditions of acute acinar cell stress.

6.5 Mice deficient in pancreatic autophagy: a new model for human CP

The present study highlighted, for the first time, the central role of Atg5-dependent autophagy in pancreatic acinar cell homeostasis. *A5* mice proceeded form early inflammation and tissue necrosis to chronic fibrosis and atrophy, covering the entire disease spectrum and exhibiting multiple similarities with the spontaneous disease in humans. Of note, p62/Nqo1/p53, damaged mitochondria, and ER stress could be detected in pancreatic tissue from both *A5* and human CP-tissues, emphasizing relevance of the pathway for the disease in humans. Moreover, treatment of *A5* mice at a stage where acinar cells exhibited the highest degree of cell stress prevented CP-formation. Figure 30 summarizes the results of the present study, proposing a model for CP-development in mice.

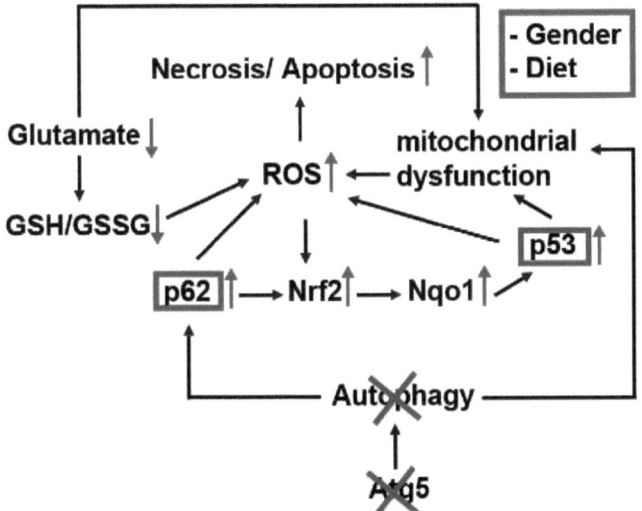

Figure 30. Signaling pathways underlying acinar cell necrosis and/or apoptosis in A5 mice. See text for details. In A5 mice Atg5 and autophagy are crossed out illustrating the blockade in autophagic signaling. Genetic knockout of Sqstm1 (i.e., p62) and Trp53 (i.e., p53) is indicated by the blue boxes; up- and downregulation of proteins, metabolites, and pathways is indicated by red and blue arrows, respectively; effect of gender and diet is highlighted by the red box.

To date, only few clinical studies were able to demonstrate a beneficial effect of antioxidants in AP[75]. Malnutrition and nutrient deficiency are known effects of CP and supplementation of certain nutrients, including fat soluble vitamins (e.g., Vitamin E), has been suggested as therapeutic option[76], but further studies are warranted. The results presented herein provide not only a model for human CP, but also suggest possible approaches for the study of therapeutic strategies.

7 SUMMARY

The central focus of the present study was to analyze the role of autophagy in pancreatic physiology and disease. Autophagy constitutes a homeostatic mechanism that plays a central role in the regulation of cellular metabolism and survival. Defective autophagy has been described in multiple degenerative and inflammatory diseases. Autophagy has also been suggested to play a role in pancreatitis, but results are contradictory.

To elucidate the importance of autophagy in exocrine pancreatic physiology, pancreas-specific *Atg5*-knockout mice were characterized in detail. Moreover, mice were treated with specific diets to study the effect of dietary composition and anti-oxidants on phenotype development. Finally, the murine pancreatic phenotype was compared to pancreata from human patients with chronic pancreatitis (CP).

Loss of pancreas-specific Atg5-dependent autophagy in mice resulted in atrophic CP, with a significantly higher frequency in males than in females. Loss of *Atg5* initiated pancreatic inflammation, necrosis, acinar-to-ductal metaplasia, and acinar cell hypertrophy, ultimately leading to tissue atrophy and degeneration. Transcriptomics and metabolomics exposed excessive reactive oxygen species and insufficient glutamate-dependent metabolic pathways as phenotype determinants. Moreover, loss of autophagy resulted in accumulation of p62, endoplasmic reticulum stress, and damaged mitochondria, further aggravated by p62/Nqo1/p53 feed-forward-signaling. Experimental acute pancreatitis was also greatly aggravated suggesting compromised acinar cell stress. Remarkably, dietary antioxidants, especially in combination with palm oil-derived fatty acids, blocked progression to CP and pancreatic acinar atrophy. Furthermore, several morphological and biochemical similarities with human CP could be identified.

Thus, the present study provides the first genetic mouse model that closely mimics human CP and proposes potential avenues for therapy.

8 REFERENCES

1. Moscat, J. & Diaz-Meco, M.T. p62: a versatile multitasker takes on cancer. *Trends in biochemical sciences* **37**, 230-236 (2012).
2. Kolodecik, T., Shugrue, C., Ashat, M. & Thrower, E.C. Risk factors for pancreatic cancer: underlying mechanisms and potential targets. *Frontiers in physiology* **4**, 415 (2013).
3. Yang, Z. & Klionsky, D.J. Eaten alive: a history of macroautophagy. *Nature cell biology* **12**, 814-822 (2010).
4. Lamb, C.A., Yoshimori, T. & Tooze, S.A. The autophagosome: origins unknown, biogenesis complex. *Nature reviews. Molecular cell biology* **14**, 759-774 (2013).
5. Mizushima, N. & Komatsu, M. Autophagy: renovation of cells and tissues. *Cell* **147**, 728-741 (2011).
6. Kroemer, G., Marino, G. & Levine, B. Autophagy and the integrated stress response. *Molecular cell* **40**, 280-293 (2010).
7. Johansen, T. & Lamark, T. Selective autophagy mediated by autophagic adapter proteins. *Autophagy* **7**, 279-296 (2011).
8. Birgisdottir, A.B., Lamark, T. & Johansen, T. The LIR motif - crucial for selective autophagy. *Journal of cell science* **126**, 3237-3247 (2013).
9. Giordano, S., Darley-Usmar, V. & Zhang, J. Autophagy as an essential cellular antioxidant pathway in neurodegenerative disease. *Redox biology* **2**, 82-90 (2014).
10. White, E. Deconvoluting the context-dependent role for autophagy in cancer. *Nature reviews. Cancer* **12**, 401-410 (2012).

11. Park, I., et al. Phosphotyrosine-independent binding of a 62-kDa protein to the src homology 2 (SH2) domain of p56lck and its regulation by phosphorylation of Ser-59 in the lck unique N-terminal region. *Proceedings of the National Academy of Sciences of the United States of America* **92**, 12338-12342 (1995).
12. Komatsu, M., Kageyama, S. & Ichimura, Y. p62/SQSTM1/A170: physiology and pathology. *Pharmacological research : the official journal of the Italian Pharmacological Society* **66**, 457-462 (2012).
13. Duran, A., et al. p62 is a key regulator of nutrient sensing in the mTORC1 pathway. *Molecular cell* **44**, 134-146 (2011).
14. Komatsu, M., et al. Homeostatic levels of p62 control cytoplasmic inclusion body formation in autophagy-deficient mice. *Cell* **131**, 1149-1163 (2007).
15. Duran, A., et al. The signaling adaptor p62 is an important NF-kappaB mediator in tumorigenesis. *Cancer cell* **13**, 343-354 (2008).
16. Ling, J., et al. KrasG12D-induced IKK2/beta/NF-kappaB activation by IL-1alpha and p62 feedforward loops is required for development of pancreatic ductal adenocarcinoma. *Cancer cell* **21**, 105-120 (2012).
17. Mathew, R., et al. Autophagy suppresses tumorigenesis through elimination of p62. *Cell* **137**, 1062-1075 (2009).
18. Inami, Y., et al. Persistent activation of Nrf2 through p62 in hepatocellular carcinoma cells. *The Journal of cell biology* **193**, 275-284 (2011).
19. Riley, B.E., et al. Ubiquitin accumulation in autophagy-deficient mice is dependent on the Nrf2-mediated stress response pathway: a potential role for protein aggregation in autophagic substrate selection. *The Journal of cell biology* **191**, 537-552 (2010).
20. Pandol, S.J. in *The Exocrine Pancreas* (San Rafael (CA), 2010).

21. Yadav, D. & Lowenfels, A.B. The epidemiology of pancreatitis and pancreatic cancer. *Gastroenterology* **144**, 1252-1261 (2013).
22. Frossard, J.L., Steer, M.L. & Pastor, C.M. Acute pancreatitis. *Lancet* **371**, 143-152 (2008).
23. Forsmark, C.E. Management of chronic pancreatitis. *Gastroenterology* **144**, 1282-1291 e1283 (2013).
24. Gukovskaya, A.S. & Gukovsky, I. Autophagy and pancreatitis. *American journal of physiology. Gastrointestinal and liver physiology* **303**, G993-G1003 (2012).
25. Gukovsky, I., Li, N., Todoric, J., Gukovskaya, A. & Karin, M. Inflammation, autophagy, and obesity: common features in the pathogenesis of pancreatitis and pancreatic cancer. *Gastroenterology* **144**, 1199-1209 e1194 (2013).
26. Hernandez-Gea, V., *et al.* Endoplasmic reticulum stress induces fibrogenic activity in hepatic stellate cells through autophagy. *Journal of hepatology* **59**, 98-104 (2013).
27. Rickmann, M., Vaquero, E.C., Malagelada, J.R. & Molero, X. Tocotrienols induce apoptosis and autophagy in rat pancreatic stellate cells through the mitochondrial death pathway. *Gastroenterology* **132**, 2518-2532 (2007).
28. Hara, T., *et al.* Suppression of basal autophagy in neural cells causes neurodegenerative disease in mice. *Nature* **441**, 885-889 (2006).
29. Harada, H., *et al.* Deficiency of p62/Sequestosome 1 causes hyperphagia due to leptin resistance in the brain. *The Journal of neuroscience : the official journal of the Society for Neuroscience* **33**, 14767-14777 (2013).

30. Jonkers, J., et al. Synergistic tumor suppressor activity of BRCA2 and p53 in a conditional mouse model for breast cancer. *Nature genetics* **29**, 418-425 (2001).
31. Nakhai, H., et al. Ptf1a is essential for the differentiation of GABAergic and glycinergic amacrine cells and horizontal cells in the mouse retina. *Development* **134**, 1151-1160 (2007).
32. Stanger, B.Z., et al. Pten constrains centroacinar cell expansion and malignant transformation in the pancreas. *Cancer cell* **8**, 185-195 (2005).
33. Muzumdar, M.D., Tasic, B., Miyamichi, K., Li, L. & Luo, L. A global double-fluorescent Cre reporter mouse. *Genesis* **45**, 593-605 (2007).
34. Mizushima, N., Yamamoto, A., Matsui, M., Yoshimori, T. & Ohsumi, Y. In vivo analysis of autophagy in response to nutrient starvation using transgenic mice expressing a fluorescent autophagosome marker. *Molecular biology of the cell* **15**, 1101-1111 (2004).
35. Demir, I.E., et al. Neuronal plasticity in chronic pancreatitis is mediated via the neurturin/GFRalpha2 axis. *American journal of physiology. Gastrointestinal and liver physiology* **303**, G1017-1028 (2012).
36. Schmidt, E.S., F.W. Methods of Enzymantic Analysis. *Verlag Chemie, Weinheim*, 216-227 (1983).
37. Folch, J., Lees, M. & Sloane Stanley, G.H. A simple method for the isolation and purification of total lipides from animal tissues. *The Journal of biological chemistry* **226**, 497-509 (1957).
38. Wiswedel, I., Gardemann, A., Storch, A., Peter, D. & Schild, L. Degradation of phospholipids by oxidative stress--exceptional significance of cardiolipin. *Free radical research* **44**, 135-145 (2010).

39. Pope, S., Land, J.M. & Heales, S.J. Oxidative stress and mitochondrial dysfunction in neurodegeneration; cardiolipin a critical target? *Biochimica et biophysica acta* **1777**, 794-799 (2008).
40. Hashimoto, D., *et al.* Involvement of autophagy in trypsinogen activation within the pancreatic acinar cells. *The Journal of cell biology* **181**, 1065-1072 (2008).
41. Witt, H., *et al.* Variants in CPA1 are strongly associated with early onset chronic pancreatitis. *Nature genetics* **45**, 1216-1220 (2013).
42. Criscimanna, A., *et al.* Duct cells contribute to regeneration of endocrine and acinar cells following pancreatic damage in adult mice. *Gastroenterology* **141**, 1451-1462, 1462 e1451-1456 (2011).
43. Jensen, J.N., *et al.* Recapitulation of elements of embryonic development in adult mouse pancreatic regeneration. *Gastroenterology* **128**, 728-741 (2005).
44. Desai, B.M., *et al.* Preexisting pancreatic acinar cells contribute to acinar cell, but not islet beta cell, regeneration. *The Journal of clinical investigation* **117**, 971-977 (2007).
45. Strobel, O., *et al.* In vivo lineage tracing defines the role of acinar-to-ductal transdifferentiation in inflammatory ductal metaplasia. *Gastroenterology* **133**, 1999-2009 (2007).
46. Hetz, C. The unfolded protein response: controlling cell fate decisions under ER stress and beyond. *Nature reviews. Molecular cell biology* **13**, 89-102 (2012).
47. Papa, S., *et al.* cAMP-dependent protein kinase regulates post-translational processing and expression of complex I subunits in mammalian cells. *Biochimica et biophysica acta* **1797**, 649-658 (2010).

48. Chicco, A.J. & Sparagna, G.C. Role of cardiolipin alterations in mitochondrial dysfunction and disease. *American journal of physiology. Cell physiology* **292**, C33-44 (2007).
49. Asher, G., Tsvetkov, P., Kahana, C. & Shaul, Y. A mechanism of ubiquitin-independent proteasomal degradation of the tumor suppressors p53 and p73. *Genes & development* **19**, 316-321 (2005).
50. Szczepanek, K., Lesnefsky, E.J. & Larner, A.C. Multi-tasking: nuclear transcription factors with novel roles in the mitochondria. *Trends in cell biology* **22**, 429-437 (2012).
51. Sundram, K., Sambanthamurthi, R. & Tan, Y.A. Palm fruit chemistry and nutrition. *Asia Pacific journal of clinical nutrition* **12**, 355-362 (2003).
52. Ong, A.S. & Goh, S.H. Palm oil: a healthful and cost-effective dietary component. *Food and nutrition bulletin* **23**, 11-22 (2002).
53. Gukovsky, I., et al. Impaired autophagy and organellar dysfunction in pancreatitis. *Journal of gastroenterology and hepatology* **27 Suppl 2**, 27-32 (2012).
54. Saluja, A.K. & Dudeja, V. Relevance of animal models of pancreatic cancer and pancreatitis to human disease. *Gastroenterology* **144**, 1194-1198 (2013).
55. Fendrich, V., et al. Hedgehog signaling is required for effective regeneration of exocrine pancreas. *Gastroenterology* **135**, 621-631 (2008).
56. Pan, H., Cai, N., Li, M., Liu, G.H. & Izpisua Belmonte, J.C. Autophagic control of cell 'stemness'. *EMBO molecular medicine* **5**, 327-331 (2013).
57. Bachmann, J., Buchler, M.W., Friess, H. & Martignoni, M.E. Cachexia in patients with chronic pancreatitis and pancreatic

cancer: impact on survival and outcome. *Nutrition and cancer* **65**, 827-833 (2013).
58. Lerch, M.M., Halangk, W. & Mayerle, J. Preventing pancreatitis by protecting the mitochondrial permeability transition pore. *Gastroenterology* **144**, 265-269 (2013).
59. Gerasimenko, O.V. & Gerasimenko, J.V. Mitochondrial function and malfunction in the pathophysiology of pancreatitis. *Pflugers Archiv : European journal of physiology* **464**, 89-99 (2012).
60. Gukovsky, I., Pandol, S.J. & Gukovskaya, A.S. Organellar dysfunction in the pathogenesis of pancreatitis. *Antioxidants & redox signaling* **15**, 2699-2710 (2011).
61. Braganza, J.M., Lee, S.H., McCloy, R.F. & McMahon, M.J. Chronic pancreatitis. *Lancet* **377**, 1184-1197 (2011).
62. Lee, J., Giordano, S. & Zhang, J. Autophagy, mitochondria and oxidative stress: cross-talk and redox signalling. *The Biochemical journal* **441**, 523-540 (2012).
63. Santos, C.X., Tanaka, L.Y., Wosniak, J. & Laurindo, F.R. Mechanisms and implications of reactive oxygen species generation during the unfolded protein response: roles of endoplasmic reticulum oxidoreductases, mitochondrial electron transport, and NADPH oxidase. *Antioxidants & redox signaling* **11**, 2409-2427 (2009).
64. Fransen, M., Nordgren, M., Wang, B. & Apanasets, O. Role of peroxisomes in ROS/RNS-metabolism: implications for human disease. *Biochimica et biophysica acta* **1822**, 1363-1373 (2012).
65. Newsholme, P., Procopio, J., Lima, M.M., Pithon-Curi, T.C. & Curi, R. Glutamine and glutamate--their central role in cell metabolism and function. *Cell biochemistry and function* **21**, 1-9 (2003).

66. Lin, T.C., *et al.* Autophagy: resetting glutamine-dependent metabolism and oxygen consumption. *Autophagy* **8**, 1477-1493 (2012).
67. Lewis, K.N., Mele, J., Hayes, J.D. & Buffenstein, R. Nrf2, a guardian of healthspan and gatekeeper of species longevity. *Integrative and comparative biology* **50**, 829-843 (2010).
68. Taguchi, K., *et al.* Keap1 degradation by autophagy for the maintenance of redox homeostasis. *Proceedings of the National Academy of Sciences of the United States of America* **109**, 13561-13566 (2012).
69. Pani, G., Koch, O.R. & Galeotti, T. The p53-p66shc-Manganese Superoxide Dismutase (MnSOD) network: a mitochondrial intrigue to generate reactive oxygen species. *The international journal of biochemistry & cell biology* **41**, 1002-1005 (2009).
70. Lista, P., Straface, E., Brunelleschi, S., Franconi, F. & Malorni, W. On the role of autophagy in human diseases: a gender perspective. *Journal of cellular and molecular medicine* **15**, 1443-1457 (2011).
71. Giergiel, M., Lopucki, M., Stachowicz, N. & Kankofer, M. The influence of age and gender on antioxidant enzyme activities in humans and laboratory animals. *Aging clinical and experimental research* **24**, 561-569 (2012).
72. Jiang, F., *et al.* Comparison of antioxidative and antifibrotic effects of alpha-tocopherol with those of tocotrienol-rich fraction in a rat model of chronic pancreatitis. *Pancreas* **40**, 1091-1096 (2011).
73. Gonzalez, A.M., *et al.* Assessment of the protective effects of oral tocotrienols in arginine chronic-like pancreatitis. *American journal of physiology. Gastrointestinal and liver physiology* **301**, G846-855 (2011).

74. Shin-Kang, S., *et al.* Tocotrienols inhibit AKT and ERK activation and suppress pancreatic cancer cell proliferation by suppressing the ErbB2 pathway. *Free radical biology & medicine* **51**, 1164-1174 (2011).
75. Hackert, T. & Werner, J. Antioxidant therapy in acute pancreatitis: experimental and clinical evidence. *Antioxidants & redox signaling* **15**, 2767-2777 (2011).
76. Rajesh, G., Girish, B.N., Vaidyanathan, K. & Balakrishnan, V. Diet, nutrient deficiency and chronic pancreatitis. *Tropical gastroenterology : official journal of the Digestive Diseases Foundation* **34**, 68-73 (2013).

9 ABBREVIATIONS

AP	Acute pancreatitis
Atg	Autophagy related
bp	Base pairs
BrdU	Bromodeoxyuridine
C II	Respiratory complex II
C IV	Respiratory complex IV
cDNA	Complementary DNA
CL	Cardiolipin
CP	Chronic pancreatitis
Da	Dalton
ER	Endoplasmic reticulum
ERK	Extracellular signal-related protein kinase
GLDH	Glutamate dehydrogenase
GSH	Glutathione
H&E	Hematoxylin and eosin
IPGTT	Intraperitoneal glucose tolerance test
NAC	N-acetylcysteine
NFkB	nuclear factor 'kappa-light-chain enhancer' of activated B-cells
Nfe2l2	Nuclear factor (erythroid-derived 2)-like 2
POD	Palm oil diet
qRT-PCR	Quantitative real time polymerase chain reaction
ROS	Reactive oxygen species
SD	Standard diet
TCA	Tricarboxylic acid
Trp53	Transformation related protein 53
UPR	Unfolded protein response
Xbp1	X-box binding protein 1

10 ACKNOWLEDGEMENTS

First of all, I would like to thank PD Dr. med. Hana Algül for accepting me as a graduate student. I am deeply grateful for the opportunity he gave me to perform research, highly relevant for human diseases in one of the most renowned hospitals of Munich. Dr. Algül provided me with excellent supervision, continuous support, and helpful discussions. Most importantly however, he enabled me to develop my own ideas and research plans, a trait critically required in the repertoire of every graduate student. I also thank Prof. Dr. med. Christos S. Mantzoros, who supported me during my doctoral research and beyond with ideas, knowledge and trust. Moreover, I thank Univ.-Prof. Dr. med. Roland M. Schmid, who along with Dr. Algül opened the doors for my doctoral studies at the TUM.

Continuing, I want to express my gratitude to all the members of my laboratory including Marina, Jiaoyu, Song, Angelika, Sonja, Matthias, Magda, Patrick, Karen, Chantal, and Viktoria. I thank you for the friendly, creative atmosphere, the helpful discussions, and the great support. Especially, I would like to thank Marina. As a postdoc she closely supervised my project, contributing significantly with thoughtful scientific ideas, multiple suggestions, and productive hard work. I am grateful for her interest in my project, her continuous readiness for discussions, and her patience and resourcefulness in trying out new research avenues.

Additionally, I want to express my gratitude to Prof. Dr. med. vet. Jörg M. Steiner. As a visiting professor to our laboratory he patiently reviewed in great detail my publication and doctoral thesis, giving superb feedback and insightful suggestions. Most importantly, his expertise in statistics greatly supported analysis of results and deepened my knowledge in the field.

Finally, I want to thank all my family and friends. I am especially grateful to my mother, father, grandmother and godfather for educating me in multiple scholarly and non-scholarly fields, their assurance during all times, their faith in me, and their never-ending support. Thank you for enriching my background and creating an environment where new ideas can always be fostered and realized.

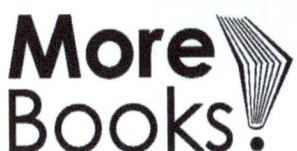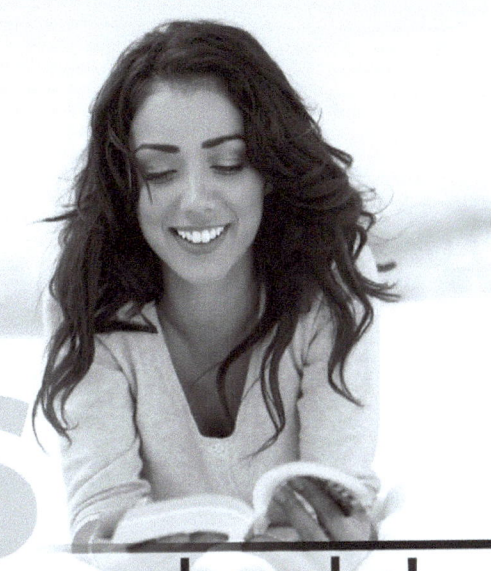

I want morebooks!

Buy your books fast and straightforward online - at one of the world's fastest growing online book stores! Environmentally sound due to Print-on-Demand technologies.

Buy your books online at
www.get-morebooks.com

Kaufen Sie Ihre Bücher schnell und unkompliziert online – auf einer der am schnellsten wachsenden Buchhandelsplattformen weltweit!
Dank Print-On-Demand umwelt- und ressourcenschonend produziert.

Bücher schneller online kaufen
www.morebooks.de

OmniScriptum Marketing DEU GmbH
Heinrich-Böcking-Str. 6-8
D - 66121 Saarbrücken
Telefax: +49 681 93 81 567-9

info@omniscriptum.com
www.omniscriptum.com

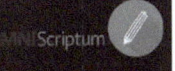

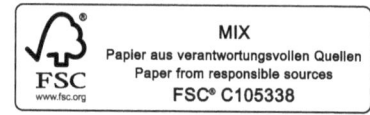

Printed by Books on Demand GmbH, Norderstedt / Germany